Rapid
Differential
Diagnosis

SABUHI KHAN
21360 MARSH CREEK DR
ASHBURN VA 20148-4023

DM78618

D1372545

RAPID
DIFFERENTIAL
DIAGNOSIS

A–Z of Symptoms, Signs and Laboratory Test Results in Medicine

Amir H. Sam
Royal Free and University College Medical School,
University College London
London

EDITORIAL ADVISOR
H.L.C. Beynon
Consultant General Physician and Rheumatologist
Royal Free and University College Medical School,
University College London
London

SERIES EDITOR
Amir H. Sam

Blackwell
Publishing

© 2003 by Blackwell Publishing Ltd
Blackwell Publishing, Inc., 350 Main Street, Malden, Massachusetts
    02148–5018, USA
Blackwell Publishing Ltd, 9600 Garsington Road, Oxford OX4 2DQ, UK
Blackwell Publishing Asia Pty Ltd, 550 Swanston Street, Carlton,
    Victoria 3053, Australia

The right of the Author to be identified as the Author of this Work has
been asserted in accordance with the Copyright, Designs and Patents Act
1988.

All rights reserved. No part of this publication may be reproduced,
stored in a retrieval system, or transmitted, in any form or by any means,
electronic, mechanical, photocopying, recording or otherwise, except as
permitted by the UK Copyright, Designs and Patents Act 1988, without
the prior permission of the publisher.

First published 2003

Library of Congress Cataloging-in-Publication Data
Sam, Amir H.
Rapid differential diagnosis: A-Z of symptoms, signs, and
laboratory test results in medicine/Amir H. Sam; editorial
advisor, H.L.C. Beynon.
        p.; cm.
    ISBN 1-4051-1097-X
    1. Diagnosis, Differential—Handbooks, manuals, etc.
    [DNLM: 1. Diagnosis, Differential—Handbooks. 2. Signs and
    Symptoms—Handbooks. 3. Laboratory Techniques and
    Procedures—Handbooks. WB 39 S187r 2003] I. Title.
    RC71.5.S25 2003
    616.07′5—dc21   2003001431

ISBN 1–4051–1097X

A catalogue record for this title is available from the British Library

Set in 7½ / 9½pt Frutiger by Kolam Information Services Pvt. Ltd., India
Printed and bound in the United Kingdom by TJ International Ltd,
    Padstow

Commissioning Editor: Vicki Noyes
Editorial Assistant: Nicola Ulyatt
Production Editor: Jonathan Rowley
Production Controller: Kate Charman

For further information on Blackwell Publishing, visit our website:
http://www.blackwellpublishing.com

Contents

Foreword

This book is a collection of the differential diagnoses of the cases presented at the Royal Free Hospital Morning Report during the period 2000–2002. Those who have studied or worked at the Royal Free Hospital remember the Morning Report as a very enjoyable and valuable learning opportunity. In these medical meetings attended by several members of the consultant body, different consultant physicians and their teams discuss various medical presentations and their causes.

The aim of *Rapid Differential Diagnosis* is to provide possible explanations for a range of symptoms, signs and laboratory test results which medical students and doctors may encounter during their study and clinical practice.

Although not exhaustive, we hope that you find this book useful in your everyday practice as well as in revising for medical examinations.

H.L.C. Beynon
January 2003

List of abbreviations

ACE	angiotensin-converting enzyme
ACTH	adrenocorticotropic hormone
AF	atrial fibrillation
ANA	antinuclear antibody
ANCA	antineutrophil cytoplasmic antibody
APTT	activated partial thromboplastin time
ARDS	acute respiratory distress syndrome
ASD	atrial septal defect
AV	atrioventricular
BPH	benign prostatic hypertrophy
CCF	congestive cardiac failure
CEA	carcinoembryonic antigen
CK	creatine kinase
CLL	chronic lymphocytic leukaemia
CMV	cytomegalovirus
CO	carbon monoxide
COPD	chronic obstructive pulmonary disorder
CRH	corticotrophin-releasing hormone
CSF	cerebrospinal fluid
CVA	cerebrovascular accident
CVS	cardiovascular system
D&C	dilatation and curettage
DAX1	dosage-sensitive sex reversal-adrenal hypoplasia gene on the X chromosome, gene 1
DIC	disseminated intravascular coagulation
DIDMOAD	diabetes insipidus, diabetes mellitus, optic atrophy, deafness
DKA	diabetic ketoacidosis
DVT	deep venous thrombosis
EBV	Epstein–Barr virus
EDTA	ethylenediaminetetraacetic acid
FSH	follicle stimulating hormone
γ-GT	gamma-glutamyl transpeptidase
G6PD	glucose-6-phosphate dehydrogenase
GGT	gamma-glutamyl transpeptidase
GnRH	gonadotropin-releasing hormone
GORD	gastroesophageal reflux disease
GTN	glyceryl trinitrate
HBV	hepatitis B virus
hCG	human chorionic gonadotropin
HCV	hepatitis C virus
HGPRT	hypoxanthine-guanine phosphoribosyl transferase
HIV	human immunodeficiency virus
HOCM	hypertrophic obstructive cardiomyopathy
HSV	herpes simplex virus
HUS	haemolytic uraemic syndrome
IBD	inflammatory bowel disease
INR	international normalized ratio
IVC	inferior vena cava
LH	luteinizing hormone
MELAS	mitochondrial encephalopathy, lactic acidosis and stroke-like episodes

MEN	multiple endocrine neoplasia
MI	myocardial infarction
MS	multiple sclerosis
MTHFR	methylene tetrahydrofolate reductase
MTP	metatarsophalangeal
OCP	oral contraceptive pill
PAN	polyarteritis nodosa
PCOS	polycystic ovary syndrome
PDA	patent ductus arteriosus
PLAP	placental-like alkaline phosphatase
PSA	prostate-specific antigen
PTH	parathyroid hormone
SAPHO	synovitis, acne, palmoplantar pustulosis, hyperostosis, osteitis
SCC	squamous cell carcinoma
SIADH	syndrome of inappropriate ADH
SLE	systemic lupus erythematosus
SVT	supraventricular tachycardia
TB	tuberculosis
TIA	transient ischaemic attack
TSH	thyroid stimulating hormone
TT	thrombin time
TTP	thrombotic thrombocytopenic purpura
UMN	upper motor neurone
UTI	urinary tract infection
VSD	ventricular septal defect
VT	ventricular tachycardia
VZV	varicella zoster virus

A

Abdominal pain

Epigastric

Peptic ulcer
Pancreatitis
Reflux oesophagitis
Acute gastritis
Malignancy: gastric, pancreatic
Pain from adjacent areas: See RUQ, central abdominal pain, cardiac/pulmonary/
  pleural pathology, e.g. MI, pericarditis, pneumonia
Functional disorders: non-ulcer dyspepsia, irritable bowel syndrome

Right upper quadrant (RUQ)

Gall bladder pathology: cholecystitis (usually related to gallstones, occasionally
  may be acalculous), biliary colic, cholangitis
Liver pathology: hepatitis, hepatomegaly (congestive, e.g. in congestive cardiac
  failure, Budd–Chiari syndrome), hepatic tumours, hepatic/subphrenic
  abscess
Pain from adjacent areas: See Epigastric (e.g. pancreatitis, peptic ulcer), RIF, Loin
  pain, pulmonary/pleural pathology, e.g. pneumonia, pulmonary infarction
Appendicitis, e.g. in a pregnant woman
Colonic cancer (hepatic flexure)
Herpes zoster

Right iliac fossa (RIF)

Gastrointestinal: appendicitis, mesenteric adenitis (Yersinia, in children), Meckel's
  diverticulum (in children), inflammatory bowel disease, colonic cancer,
  constipation, irritable bowel syndrome
Reproductive: Females: Mittelschmerz (ovulation), ovarian cyst torsion/rupture/
  haemorrhage, ectopic pregnancy, salpingitis/pelvic inflammatory disease,
  endometriosis. Males: seminal vesiculitis, cancer in undescended testis
Renal: UTI, ureteric colic (renal stones)
Pain from adjacent areas: See RUQ, suprapubic, central abdominal pain, groin
  pain, hip pathology, psoas abscess, rectus sheath haematoma, right-sided
  lobar pneumonia

Suprapubic

Urinary retention
Cystitis
Pain from adjacent areas: See RIF, LIF

Left iliac fossa (LIF)

Gastrointestinal: diverticulitis, inflammatory bowel disease, colonic cancer,
  constipation, irritable bowel syndrome
Reproductive: See RIF
Renal pain: See RIF
Pain from adjacent areas: See LUQ, suprapubic, central abdominal, hip pathology,
  psoas abscess, rectus sheath haematoma, left-sided lobar pneumonia

Left upper quadrant (LUQ)

Splenic rupture, splenic infarction (e.g. sickle cell disease), splenomegaly
Subphrenic abscess

Abdominal pain continued

Pain from adjacent areas: *See* epigastric (e.g. pancreatitis, peptic ulcer), LIF, loin pain, cardiac/pulmonary/pleural pathology, e.g. MI, pericarditis, pneumonia, empyema, pulmonary infarction

Colonic cancer (splenic flexure)

Herpes zoster

Central abdominal (periumbilical)

Gastrointestinal: intestinal obstruction, early appendicitis, gastroenteritis

Vascular: abdominal aortic aneurysm (leaking, ruptured), mesenteric ischaemia (thrombosis, embolism, vasculitis, e.g. polyarteritis nodosa)

Medical causes, e.g. diabetic ketoacidosis, uraemia

Pain from adjacent areas, e.g. epigastric, iliac fossae

Loin pain

Infection: UTI (pyelonephritis), perinephric abscess/pyonephrosis

Obstruction, e.g. renal stones (*See* Urinary tract obstruction)

Renal carcinoma

Renal vein thrombosis

Polycystic kidney disease

Pain from vertebral column

Groin pain

Renal stones (pain radiating from loin to groin)

Testicular pain, e.g. torsion, epididymo-orchitis (pain radiating from scrotum to groin)

Hernia (inguinal)

Hip pathology

Pelvic fractures

Diffuse abdominal pain

Gastroenteritis

Peritonitis

Intestinal obstruction

Inflammatory bowel disease

Mesenteric ischaemia

Medical causes (see below)

Irritable bowel syndrome

Medical causes

CVS/Respiratory: MI, pneumonia, Bornholm's disease (Coxsackie B virus infection, rare)

Metabolic: diabetic ketoacidosis, Addisonian crisis, hypercalcaemia, uraemia, porphyria, phaeochromocytoma, lead poisoning

Neurological: Herpes zoster, tabes dorsalis

Haematological: sickle cell crisis, retroperitoneal haemorrhage (e.g. anticoagulants), lymphadenopathy

Inflammatory: vasculitis (e.g. Henoch–Schönlein purpura, polyarteritis nodosa), familial Mediterranean fever

Infections: intestinal parasites, tuberculosis, malaria, typhoid fever

Irritable bowel syndrome

Abdominal distension

Fat (obesity)

Fluid (ascites, fluid in the obstructed intestine)

Flatus (intestinal obstruction*)
Faeces
Fetus
Giant organomegaly (e.g. an ovarian cystadenoma, lymphoma)

*Small bowel: adhesions, herniae, intussusception, Crohn's disease, gallstone
   ileus, foreign body, tumour, tuberculosis. Large bowel: cancer, volvulus,
   diverticulitis, faeces.

Abdominal masses
See Masses and swellings

Abdominal wall veins, dilated
Caput medusae (portal hypertension)
Inferior vena cava obstruction

Acanthosis nigricans
Malignancy: oesophagus, stomach, large bowel, bladder, kidney
Insulin resistance: diabetes mellitus, PCOS, steroids
Acromegaly
Prader–Willi syndrome

Acanthocytosis
Artifact (blood collected in EDTA tube)
Abetalipoproteinaemia (associated with retinitis pigmentosa, neurological
   deficits)
Anorexia
Liver failure
Chronic renal failure
Hyposplenism
Hypothyroidism
Chorea–acanthocytosis syndrome

ACE (Angiotensin-converting enzyme), ↑
Sarcoidosis
TB
Lymphoma
Asbestosis
Silicosis

Acid phosphatase, ↑
Prostate cancer
Paget's disease of bone
Lysosomal storage disease, e.g. Gaucher's disease
Thrombocythaemia

Acidosis
Metabolic
Normal anion gap
↓ HCO_3^- GI loss: diarrhoea, fistula (biliary, intestinal, pancreatic), ileostomy,
   ureterosigmoidostomy
   Renal loss: renal tubular acidosis (type 2), renal tubular damage (e.g. drugs/
   heavy metals), hyperparathyroidism, acetazolamide
↑ H^+ Renal tubular acidosis (1 & 4), ammonium chloride ingestion

Acidosis continued

High anion gap

Ketoacidosis: diabetes mellitus, excess alcohol, starvation

Lactic acidosis:

    Tissue hypoxia, e.g. shock (haemorrhagic/septic), severe exercise, severe anaemia

    Drugs: metformin, ethanol, methanol, ethylene glycol, zidovudine

    D-Lactic acidosis (short gut syndrome)

    Leukaemia

    Lymphoma

    Liver failure

    Glucose-6-phosphatase deficiency, mitochondrial disorders (e.g. MELAS)

Renal failure

Salicylate poisoning

Respiratory

CNS

Organic disease involving respiratory centre (e.g. vascular, infection, inflammation, trauma, tumour)

Drugs: opiates, benzodiazepines, barbiturates and other anaesthetic agents

Lungs

Severe asthma (uncommonly), COPD, large airway obstruction, obstructive sleep apnoea

Neuromuscular

Motor neurones: Guillain–Barré syndrome, motor neurone disease, poliomyelitis, acute porphyria

Neuromuscular junction/muscle: myasthenia gravis, muscular dystrophies, muscle relaxants, diaphagmatic paralysis

Chest wall

Severe kyphoscoliosis, severe obesity, traumatic 'flail chest'

Acute confusional state

See Delirium

Ageusia

Infection/inflammatory diseases of oral cavity

Chorda tympani injury, e.g. during surgery (unilateral anterior 2/3 of the tongue)

Radiation

See also Dysgeusia (impairment of taste)

Alanine-amino transferase (ALT)

See Liver function tests

Alkaline phosphatase

See Liver function tests

Alkalosis

Metabolic

GI loss of H$^+$

Vomiting, laxative abuse, villous adenoma, VIPoma

Renal loss of H⁺
↑↑ *Mineralocorticoid activity (stimulates H⁺ secretion):*
Hyperaldosteronism
↑↑ Glucocorticoids: Cushing's syndrome, liquorice (inhibits 11-hydroxysteroid
    dehydrogenase and ↓ glucocorticoid metabolism)

↑ Na⁺ *delivery to distal nephron*
Diuretics: thiazides and loop diuretics (also ↑ aldosterone secretion)
Bartter's syndrome, Gitelman's syndrome

Intracellular shift of H⁺
Hypokalaemia (also note that the above causes of GI/renal loss of H⁺, also induce
    K⁺ loss)

Other
Compensation for respiratory acidosis
Excessive alkali ingestion (e.g. ↑↑ sodium bicarbonate administration in treatment
    of acidotic states)
Fulminant hepatic failure (failure to synthesize urea and neutralize bicarbonate
    derived from amino acid metabolism)

Respiratory
Hyperventilation:
    Physiological (anxiety, pain, fever, pregnancy, high altitude)
    Mechanical overventilation
    Respiratory failure (type I): asthma, COPD, pneumonia, pulmonary oedema,
    pulmonary embolism, ARDS, fibrosing alveolitis, right → left shunt
    Salicylate poisoning, CO poisoning
    CNS disease (CVA, infection, tumour, trauma)
    Others: liver failure (acute), Gram −ve septicaemia

Alopecia
Non-scarring
Aging (male/female pattern baldness)
Alopecia areata
Traction, trichotillomania
Telogen effluvium: transitory ↑ in number of hairs in resting phase of the hair
    growth cycle, associated with stress, (e.g. surgery, febrile illness, childbirth, etc.)
Cutaneous diseases (e.g. psoriasis, eczema)
Drugs (cytotoxics, ciclosporin, OCPs, anticoagulants, antithyroid drugs, vitamin A/
    retinoids)
Endocrine diseases (hypopituitarism, hypo/hyperthyroidism, diabetes mellitus)
Nutritional deficiency (iron, zinc, biotin, caloric deficiency)
Congenital

Scarring
Trauma/burns
Infection: pyogenic infection, TB (lupus vulgaris), syphilis, viral (varicella, herpes
    simplex), fungal (e.g. ringworm), protozoal (Leishmaniasis), leprosy
Inflammatory disease: SLE, scleroderma, sarcoidosis
Skin disease: lichen planus, cicatricial pemphigoid, necrobiosis lipoidica, folliculitis
    decalvans

Ambiguous genitalia
See Pseudohermaphrodite

Amenorrhoea

Non-pathological: pregnancy, lactation, menopause, drugs (e.g. Depo-Provera)
Hypothalamus: starvation, anorexia, excessive exercise, weight loss, *GnRH deficiency* (isolated or part of Kallmann's syndrome)
Pituitary: hypopituitarism, hyperprolactinaemia
Ovaries: PCOS, premature ovarian failure, damage to ovaries (infection e.g. mumps, autoimmune, surgery, radiotherapy), *ovarian dysgensis (e.g. Turner's syndrome)*
Uterus/vagina: *absent uterus, imperforate hymen, transverse vaginal septum*
    Asherman's syndrome: scarring of endometrial lining 2° to infection and instrumentation, e.g. D&C
Thyroid: hypo/hyperthyroidism
Adrenals: adrenal tumours, Cushing's syndrome
Note: The causes in *italics* present only with primary amenorrhoea.

Amnesia
Acute/transient
In the presence of other cognitive deficits: acute confusional state (*See* Delirium)
Trauma (head injury)
Transient global amnesia (may be associated with migraine)
Temporal lobe epilepsy
Migraine
Transient ischaemic attack (TIA), tumours (rare)

Chronic/persistent
In the presence of other cognitive deficits (*See* Dementia)
Medial temporal lobe lesions (bilateral)
Vascular: posterior cerebral artery occlusion (bilateral)
Infection: herpes simplex encephalitis
Inflammation: limbic encephalitis (may be paraneoplastic), sarcoidosis
Tumours: midline (in the region of the third ventricle)
Toxic/metabolic: thiamine deficiency (Korsakoff's psychosis in alcoholism, hyperemesis gravidarum)

Amylase, ↑
Pancreatitis (acute)
Acute abdomen: peptic ulcer, perforation, intestinal obstruction, ruptured ectopic pregnancy
Diabetic ketoacidosis
Renal failure
Salivary gland disorders: calculi, mumps
Morphine (spasm of sphincter of Oddi)
Macroamylasaemia: amylase is complexed with another protein, e.g. immunoglobulin and its renal clearance is reduced

ANA
SLE (95%), drug-induced lupus (100%)
Systemic sclerosis (90%)
Sjögren's syndrome (80%)
Rheumatoid arthritis (60%)
Polymyositis (40%)
Polyarteritis nodosa (20%)
Other diseases: chronic active hepatitis, diabetes, Waldenström's macroglobulinaemia, myasthenia gravis
Normal population (5–8%)

Anaemia
Macrocytic
Alcohol
Folate/B_{12} deficiency
Haemolytic anaemia
Hypothyroidism
Liver disease
Myelodysplasia

Microcytic
Iron deficiency: blood loss (GI [e.g. peptic ulcer, malignancy], urogenital [e.g.
    menorrhagia, haematuria]), hookworm (Ancylostroma duodenale)
    ↓ absorption (gastrectomy, small bowel disease),
    ↑ demands (growth, pregnancy), ↓ intake (e.g. vegans)
Thalassaemia
Sideroblastic anaemia: congenital (X-linked), alcohol, drugs (isoniazid,
    chloramphenicol), lead, myelodysplasia
Lead poisoning
Anaemia of chronic disease (often normocytic, but may be microcytic)

Normocytic
Anaemia of chronic disease (chronic infection, inflammatory/connective tissue
    diseases, malignancy)
Haemolytic anaemia (may also cause macrocytic anaemia)
Hypothyroidism (may also cause macrocytic anaemia)
Pregnancy
Renal failure
Bone marrow failure

Haemolytic
Hereditary
Haemoglobinopathies: sickle cell anaemia, thalassaemia
Membrane defects: spherocytosis, elliptocytosis
Metabolic defects: pyruvate kinase deficiency, glucose-6-phosphate
    dehydrogenase deficiency

Acquired
Autoimmune: Warm antibodies (idiopathic, SLE, lymphoma, drugs, e.g.
    methyldopa), Cold antibodies (idiopathic, infections, e.g. *Mycoplasma* sp.,
    EBV, other viruses, lymphoma)
Alloimmune: Transfusion reaction, haemolytic disease of newborn
Drugs: penicillin, quinidine
Non-immune: trauma: microangiopathic haemolytic anaemia (TTP, HUS, DIC,
    malignant hypertension, pre-eclampsia), artificial heart valves, March
    haemoglobinuria
Infection: malaria, clostridia
Paroxysmal nocturnal haemoglobinuria, secondary to liver and renal disease

Aplastic
Idiopathic
Inherited: Fanconi anaemia, dyskeratosis congenita
Acquired: drugs (cytotoxics, chloramphenicol, gold, methotrexate), chemicals
    (parathion, benzene), radiation, viral infection (B19 parvovirus, HIV,
    hepatitis, measles), paroxysmal nocturnal haemoglobinuria, sepsis

ANCA
p-ANCA
Microscopic polyangiitis
Churg–Strauss disease
Also: inflammatory bowel disease, sclerosing cholangitis, biliary cirrhosis,
   autoimmune hepatitis, rheumatic autoimmune diseases

c-ANCA
Wegener's granulomatosis
Infections, e.g. amoebic colitis

Androgenization
PCOS
Congenital adrenal hyperplasia
Cushing's syndrome
Adrenal tumours

Angioid streaks
Pseudoxanthoma elasticum
Ehlers–Danlos syndrome
Paget's disease of bone
Sickle cell anaemia
Acromegaly, hypercalcaemia, lead poisoning

Angular stomatitis
See Cheilitis

Anisocoria
Physiological inequality
Unilateral miosis (*See* Miosis) or mydriasis (*See* Mydriasis)
Prosthetic eyeball

Anisocytosis
Iron deficiency
Thalassaemia
Megaloblastic anaemia

Ankle oedema
See Oedema

Annular skin lesions
Tinea corporis
Urticaria
Pityriasis rosea
Granuloma annulare
Sarcoidosis
Subacute cutaneous lupus erythematosus
Erythema annulare centrifugum
Erythema chronicum migrans
Erythema multiforme
Nummular eczema
Psoriasis
Leprosy

Anorectal pain
Anal fissure

Haemorrhoids (strangulated, thrombosed)
Perianal abscess
Perianal haematoma
Proctalgia fugax
Malignancy
Trauma
Solitary rectal ulcer

Anosmia
Nasal congestion (rhinitis), nasal polyps
Neurological: tumours on the floor of the anterior fossa (e.g. meningioma), head
    trauma, neurodegenerative diseases
Congenital: Kallmann's syndrome (anosmia and GnRH deficiency), cleft palate

Aortic regurgitation
Valve leaflet damage/abnormalities: infective endocarditis, rheumatic fever,
    trauma, bicuspid aortic valve
Aorta and valve ring dilatation: aortic dissection, aortitis (e.g. syphilis), arthritides
    (rheumatoid arthritis, seronegative arthritides, e.g. ankylosing spondylitis,
    Reiter's syndrome), ↑↑BP
Others: Marfan's syndrome, pseudoxanthoma elasticum, Ehlers–Danlos
    syndrome, osteogenesis imperfecta, inflammatory bowel disease

Aortic stenosis
Stenosis secondary to rheumatic heart disease
Calcification of a congenital bicuspid AV
Calcification/degeneration of a tricuspid AV in elderly

Apex beat
Heaving (pressure loaded)
Aortic stenosis (*See* Aortic stenosis)
Systemic hypertension

Thrusting (volume loaded)
Mitral regurgitation (*See* Mitral regurgitation)
Aortic regurgitation (*See* Aortic regurgitation)

Tapping
Mitral stenosis (*See* Mitral stenosis)

Apex beat not palpated
Obesity, muscular chest wall
Dextrocardia
COPD
L-sided pneumothorax
L-sided pleural effusion
Large pericardial effusion

Aphasia
See Dysphasia

Appetite, ↓
See Weight loss, ↓ appetite

APTT, ↑
Haemophilia
von Willebrand's disease
Liver disease
Warfarin therapy, vitamin K deficiency
Heparin
DIC

Note: APTT monitors the intrinsic pathway i.e. deficiency or inhibition of
    coagulation factors: XII, XI, IX, VIII, X, V, II, and fibrinogen

Arachnodactyly
Normal finding
Marfan's syndrome
Homocysteinuria
Ehlers–Danlos syndrome

Arm pain
Trauma, strain injury
Arthritis (See Monoarthralgia)
Neurological: cervical spinal cord compression (prolapsed disc, cervical
    spondylosis, tumours)
Brachial plexus involvement: apical lung cancer, cervical rib
Peripheral neuropathies
Carpal tunnel syndrome
Vascular: subclavian artery stenosis, arterial/venous thrombosis, embolism
Bone: tumours (primary, secondary: lung, breast, prostate, kidney, thyroid)
Referred cardiac pain
See also Shoulder pain

Arm swelling
Congenital lymphoedema (rare)
Trauma
Cellulitis
Deep venous thrombosis (DVT) (axillary vein: associated with excessive exercise,
    cervical rib)
Axillary lymph node involvement: radiotherapy, surgical excision, malignancy,
    filariasis

Arterial blood gases
Hypoxia, normal or low P_aCO_2 (respiratory failure: type 1)
Asthma
COPD
Pulmonary embolism
Pulmonary oedema
Pneumonia
Pulmonary fibrosis
R → L shunt
ARDS

Hypoxia, high P_aCO_2 (respiratory failure: type 2)
CNS:
    Organic disease involving respiratory centre (vascular, infection, inflammation,
        trauma, tumour)
    Drugs: opiates, benzodiazepines, barbiturates and other anaesthetic agents
Lungs:

Severe asthma, COPD, large airway obstruction, obstructive sleep apnoea
Neuromuscular:
    Motor neurones: Guillain–Barré syndrome, motor neurone disease,
        poliomyelitis, acute porphyria
    Neuromuscular junction/muscle: myasthenia gravis, muscular dystrophies
        muscle relaxants, diaphragmatic paralysis
Chest wall:
    Severe kyphoscoliosis, severe obesity, traumatic 'flail chest'

Arthralgia
See Monoarthralgia and Polyarthralgia

Ascites
Exudate
Malignancy (abdominal, pelvic, peritoneal mesothelioma)
Infection: e.g. TB, pyogenic
Pancreatitis
Myxoedema (hypothyroidism)
Budd–Chiari syndrome (hepatic vein obstruction), portal vein thrombosis
Chylous ascites (obstruction of lymphatics, e.g. surgery, lymphoma)

Transudate
Cirrohsis
Cardiac failure, constrictive pericarditis
Nephrotic syndrome
Rare: Meigs' syndrome (ovarian fibroma, ascites, pleural effusion), ovarian
    hyperstimulation

Aspartate-amino transferase (AST, SGOT)
See Liver function tests

AST
See Liver function tests

Asterixis
Liver failure
CO_2 retention

Ataxia
Cerebellar ataxia
Vascular: infarction, haemorrhage
Infection: varicella, cerebellar abscess, TB, toxoplasmosis, cysticercosis
Inflammation: multiple sclerosis, vasculitis
Trauma
Tumour: cerebellar haemangioblastoma, astrocytoma, metastases,
    paraneoplastic
Toxic/metabolic: alcohol, phenytoin, myxoedema
Congenital: cerebellar hypoplasia, Dandy–Walker syndrome, Arnold–Chiari
    malformation
Degenerative: multiple system atrophy
Hereditary ataxias: autosomal recessive (e.g. Friedreich's ataxia, ataxia
    telangiectasia), autosomal dominant (e.g. spinocerebellar ataxia)
Storage diseases, e.g. Niemann–Pick disease, Tay–Sachs disease, ceroid
    lipofuscinosis, metachromatic leukodystrophy, sialidosis and numerous
    other genetic/metabolic causes, e.g. Refsum disease, Wilson's disease, etc.

Ataxia continued
Sensory ataxia
Subacute combined degeneration of the cord (*See* B$_{12}$ deficiency), syphilis (tabes dorsalis), cervical myelopathy, diabetic pseudotabes

Avascular necrosis
Fracture (e.g. scaphoid, neck of femur)
Radiotherapy
Sickle cell
Steroids
Cushing's syndrome
Connective tissue diseases (e.g. rheumatoid arthritis, SLE)
Pregnancy
Pancreatitis
Alcohol
Other: Fabry's disease, Gaucher's disease; Caisson's disease (in deep-sea divers)

Axillary erythematosus rash
Seborrhoeic dermatitis
Contact dermatitis
Flexural psoriasis
Fungal infection: candidiasis, tinea
Erythrasma (*Corynebacterium* infection)

Axis deviation
Left axis deviation (LAD)
Left anterior hemiblock
MI (inferior wall)
Wolff–Parkinson–White syndrome (some types)
Ventricular tachycardia (left ventricular focus)
Obesity, pregnancy, congenital heart defects (e.g. endocardial cushion defects)

Right axis deviation (RAD)
Right ventricular hypertrophy (e.g. secondary to COPD), pulmonary embolism
MI (antero-lateral)
Wolff–Parkinson–White (left-sided accessory pathway)
Dextrocardia
Left posterior hemiblock (rare)

B

B$_{12}$ deficiency
↓ Absorption
↓ Intrinsic factor (pernicious anaemia, gastrectomy)
Terminal ileal surgery/disease (coeliac disease, Crohn's disease, tuberculosis, bacterial overgrowth, lymphoma, tropical sprue, fish tapeworm)
Drug-induced malabsorption, e.g. metformin

Other ↓ intake (vegans)
Transcobalmin deficiency (congenital), nitrous oxide (inactivates B$_{12}$)

Back pain
Trauma/fractures, strenuous activity

Younger patients (≤40 year)
Prolapsed disc, ankylosing spondylitis, spondylolisthesis

Older patients (≥40 year)
Osteoarthritis, spinal stenosis and spinal claudication, osteoporosis, Paget's disease of bone, herpes zoster

Serious causes
Infection (TB, bacterial osteomyelitis)
Malignancy (metastasis, multiple myeloma)
Cord compression

Vascular/GI/pelvic
Aortic aneurysm, peptic ulcer, pancreatic cancer, renal disease, rectal cancer, uterine tumours, pelvic inflammatory disease, endometriosis, ovarian cyst

Basophilic stippling
Pyrimidine-5′-nucleotidase deficiency
Lead poisoning (inhibition of pyrimidine-5′-nucleotidase)
Sideroblastic anaemia
Thalassaemia

Belching, bloating and flatulence
↑ Awareness of normal amount of gas
Aerophagia (habitual swallowing of large amounts of air)
Air entrapment (hepatic or splenic flexure)
Foods containing the carbohydrate raffinose, e.g. beans, cabbage, cauliflower
Malabsorption: bacterial overgrowth (small intestine), coeliac disease, biliary disease, pancreatic insufficiency, pancreatic carcinoma
Non-ulcer dyspepsia
Irritable bowel syndrome
Intolerance to lactose (and other sugars)
Inflammation around the anus (e.g. haemorrhoids) and oesophagus (e.g. oesophagitis)
Infection: Giardiasis

Blackouts
Cardiovascular (transient ↓ blood flow to the brain)
Arrhythmia: bradycardia (heart block), tachycardia
Outflow obstruction: aortic stenosis, HOCM, pulmonary embolism, pulmonary
  stenosis
Postural hypotension: hypovolaemia, autonomic neuropathy (e.g. diabetes),
  antihypertensive medication (e.g. ACE inhibitors)
MI, aortic dissection, any condition that ↓ cardiac output

Neurological
Epilepsy, stroke/transient ischaemic attack (TIA) (rarely)

Vasovagal (reflex bradycardia)
Prolonged standing esp. in warm surroundings, emotion
Other causes of vagal overactivity: micturition, cough, carotid sinus
  hypersensitivity (e.g. on shaving the neck or head-turning)
Metabolic: hypoglycaemia
Note: there is no clearcut loss of consciousness in 'drop attacks'

Blasts
Leukaemia
Myelofibrosis

Bleeding, prolonged
Platelet disorders (*see* Bleeding time)
Coagulation disorders:
  Haemophilia
  Liver disease
  Vitamin K deficiency/warfarin
  Disseminated intravascular coagulation

Bleeding time, ↑
Thrombocytopenia (*See* Thrombocytopenia)

Bloating
See Belching, bloating and flatulence

Blood film
Acanthocytes: *See* Acanthocytosis
Anisocytosis: *See* Anisocytosis
Basophilic stippling: *See* Basophilic stippling
Blasts: *See* Blasts
Burr cells: *See* Burr cells
Dimorphic blood film: *See* Dimorphic blood film
Howell–Jolly bodies: *See* Howell–Jolly bodies
Hypochromia: *See* Hypochromia
Leukoerythroblastic anaemia: *See* Leukoerythroblastic anaemia
Leukaemoid reaction: *See* Leukaemoid reaction
Normoblasts: *See* Normoblasts
Pappenheimer bodies: *See* Pappenheimer bodies
Poikilocytosis: *See* Poikilocytosis
Polychromasia: *See* Polychromasia
Reticulocytosis: *See* Reticulocytosis
Spherocytosis: *See* Spherocytosis

Target cells: *See* Target cells
Teardrop cells: *See* Teardrop cells

Blood pressure, ↑ & ↓
See under Hypertension and Hypotension

Bloody diarrhoea
See Diarrhoea

Blue nail(s)
Subungal haematoma
Melanoma
Pseudomonas infection
Wilson's disease

Blue sclerae
Pseudoxanthoma elasticum
Osteogenesis imperfecta
Ehlers–Danlos syndrome
Marfan's syndrome

Bowing of tibia
Paget's disease
Rickets
Treponemal disease: syphilis, yaws
McCune–Albright syndrome
Osteogenesis imperfecta

Bradycardia
Sleep
Physical fitness
Vasovagal attacks
Drugs: amiodarone, β-blocker, Ca^{2+} channel antagonist (e.g. verapamil), digoxin
Acute MI (Sinus node ischaemia), sick sinus syndrome
Atrioventricular block
Cushing's reflex (↑ intracranial pressure)
Hypothyroidism
Hypothermia
Obstructive jaundice

Breast lumps
Fibroadenoma
Cyst
Cancer
Fat necrosis
Galactocoele
Duct ectasia
Abscess
Non-breast lumps: lipomas, sebaceous cysts

Breast pain
Cyclical breast pain
Infection (breast abscess, mastitis)
Malignancy

Breast pain continued
Duct ectasia
Fat necrosis
Chest wall pain: costochondritis, superficial thrombophlebitis

Breath sounds, ↓
Collapse
Pleural effusion
Pneumothorax
Emphysema

Breathlessness
Acute (minutes)
Pulmonary embolism
Pneumothorax
Foreign body
Anaphylaxis
Anxiety

Subacute (hours)
Left ventricular failure (pulmonary oedema)
Asthma
COPD
Chest infection (bacterial, viral, fungal, TB)
Metabolic acidosis

Chronic (days–weeks)
Anaemia
Recurrent pulmonary emboli
Cardiac disease (heart failure, arrhythmias, valvular heart disease)
Asthma
COPD
Chest infection, bronchiectasis
Lung cancer
Pulmonary fibrosis (cryptogenic, connective tissue diseases, drugs, environmental/
    occupational lung disease)
Pulmonary hypertension
Hepatorenal syndrome
Cirrhotic hydrothorax
Neuromuscular disorders, chest wall deformities

Bronchial breathing
Consolidation (pneumonia)
Above pleural effusion
Abscess
Lung cancer
Fibrosis

Bulbar and pseudobulbar palsy
Bulbar palsy: cranial nerves (IX, X, XII) lesions at three different levels:
Nuclei (brainstem): vascular, infection (e.g. polio encephalitis), syringobulbia,
    tumour
Nerve: motor neurone disease, meningeal infiltration, Guillain–Barré syndrome
Muscle: myasthenia gravis, muscular dystrophy, polymyositis

Pseudobulbar palsy: bilateral UMN lesions to the lower brainstem
Multiple sclerosis
Motor neurone disease
Malignancy
Vascular disease (involving both hemispheres)
Extrapyramidal disease

Bullous skin lesions
Bites (e.g. insect/snake), burns
Infections: impetigo, cellulitis, viral (VZV, HSV, coxsackie), fungal (tinea pedis, 'id' reaction), scabies
Pemphigus, pemphigoid
Pregnancy: herpes gestationis
Porphyria cutanea tarda
Dermatitis herpetiformis (associated with coeliac disease)
Diabetes
Drugs
Eczema (hand and foot)
Erythema multiforme
Epidermolysis bullosa congenita, epidermolysis bullosa acquisita (associated with inflammatory bowel disease, internal malignancy, amyloidosis)

Bundle branch blocks, left and right
Left bundle branch block (LBBB)
Ischaemic heart disease
Cardiomyopathy
Left ventricular hypertrophy (aortic stenosis, hypertension)
Conduction system fibrosis

Right bundle branch block (RBBB)
Ischaemic heart disease
Cardiomyopathy
Massive pulmonary embolism
Atrial septal defect, Ebstein's anomaly

Burr cells
Stomach cancer
Renal failure
Pyruvate kinase deficiency
Post-transfusion

C

Cachexia
Malnutrition, eating disorders
Malignancy
Infection (e.g. TB, Cryptosporidium in AIDS)
Congestive cardiac failure
Alzheimer's disease

Café-au-lait spots
Neurofibromatosis
Tuberous sclerosis
McCune–Albright syndrome
Fanconi anaemia

Calf swelling/pain
Deep venous thrombosis
Cellulitis, necrotizing fasciitis
Baker's cyst rupture
Trauma, compartment syndrome
Ruptured popliteal aneurysm
Ruptured gastrocnemius

Candidiasis
Diabetes mellitus
Drugs: broad-spectrum antibiotics, immunosuppressants, steroids
Extremes of age
HIV
Malignancy
Pregnancy
Iron deficiency (severe)
Chronic mucocutaneous candidiasis

Carotenaemia
Excess carrots, oranges, mangoes
Hypothyroidism
Lipoproteinaemia

Carpal tunnel syndrome
Idiopathic
Amyloidosis (e.g. β2-microglobulin related amyloidosis in chronic renal
    failure)
Acromegaly
Myxoedema
Pregnancy, oral contraception (fluid retention)
Obesity
Osteoarthritis
Rheumatoid arthritis
Diabetes mellitus
Fracture (local deformity)
Trauma, manual occupations
(↑ Triglycerides can cause dysaethesias similar to carpal tunnel syndrome)

CEA
See Tumour markers

Cerebellar signs
See Ataxia

Charcot's joint
Diabetes mellitus
Syphilis (tabes dorsalis)
Syringomyelia
Leprosy
Others: yaws, progressive sensory neuropathy, Charcot–Marie–Tooth disease, neurofibromatosis (pressure on sensory nerve roots)

Cheilitis (angular stomatitis)
Iron deficiency anaemia
Riboflavin deficiency
Candidiasis
Contact dermatitis (e.g. lipsticks, pen-sucking)
Lip-sucking
Overclosure of the mouth (e.g. without teeth or with dentures)

Cherry red spot
Central retinal artery occlusion (thrombosis, embolus, spasm, giant cell arteritis)
Lysosomal storage diseases: sialidosis, Tay–Sachs disease, Niemann–Pick disease, metachromatic leukodystrophy
CO poisoning

Chest pain
Cardiac/large vessels: angina pectoris, myocardial infarction, pericarditis, aortic dissection, rupture of thoracic aortic aneurysm, bleeding into an atheroma
Respiratory: pulmonary embolism, pneumothorax, pneumonia, connective tissue diseases (e.g. SLE)
Gastrointestinal: reflux oesophagitis, oesophageal spasm, hiatus hernia, peptic ulcer, pancreatitis
Musculoskeletal: Teitze's syndrome (costochondritis), fractured rib, Bornholm's disease (Coxackie B virus infection, rare)
Neurological: herpes zoster, nerve root compression

Pleuritic chest pain
Pulmonary embolism
Pneumothorax
Pneumonia
Pericarditis
Connective tissue disease
Malignancy involving pleura, pathology under the diaphragm

Chest X-ray
Bilateral hilar lymphadenopathy
TB
Sarcoidosis
Lymphoma
Others: bronchial carcinoma, metastatic tumours, recurrent chest infections, AIDS, berylliosis, silicosis

Chest X-ray continued
Cavitating lung lesions
Abscess
Tumour (particularly squamous cell carcinoma)
Infarct

Coin lesions
Tumours: bronchial carcinoma, metastatic deposit, e.g. breast cancer, renal cell
  carcinoma, hamartoma, adenoma, fibroma
Infection: pneumonia, TB, abscess, hydatid cyst
Infarction
Encysted pleural effusion
Rheumatoid nodule
Vasculitides (e.g. Wegener's granulomatosis)
AV malformation

Airspace/alveolar shadows
Pus (consolidation)
Fluid (pulmonary oedema)
Blood (pulmonary haemorrhage)
Cells (lymphangitis carcinomatosis, alveolar cell carcinoma)

Reticulonodular shadows
Pulmonary fibrosis:
Cryptogenic fibrosing alveolitis
Connective tissue diseases: scleroderma, SLE, sarcoidosis, rheumatoid arthritis,
  ankylosing spondylitis
Drugs (amiodarone, busulphan, bleomycin, nitrofurantoin), radiation
Extrinsic allergic alveolitis (e.g. farmers' lung, bird fancier's lung, malt worker's
  lung)
Pneumoconioses (coal workers' pneumoconiosis, asbestosis, silicosis, berylliosis)

Reticulonodular shadows (classified according to the lung zones in which they commonly occur)
Upper zone: allergic bronchopulmoary aspergillosis, radiation, extrinsic allergic
  alveolitis, ankylosing spondylitis, sarcoidosis, TB (commonest)
Middle zone: sarcoidosis
Lower zone: cryptogenic fibrosing alveolitis, drugs, asbestosis, rheumatoid
  arthritis, scleroderma

White hemithorax
Large pleural effusion
Pneumonectomy
Congenital absence of lung/extensive hypoplasia
Collapse

Cheyne–Stokes respiration
Brainstem lesions or compression (e.g. stroke, ↑ intracranial pressure)
Left ventricular failure
Morphine

Chondrocalcinosis/pseudogout
Osteoarthritis
Excess divalent ions: copper (Wilson's disease), iron (haemochromatosis), calcium
  (hyperparathyroidism)

Acromegaly
Ochronosis (alkaptonuria)
Hypomagnesaemia
Hypophosphataemia

Chorea
Huntington's disease
Wilson's disease
Oral contraception
Pregnancy
Polycythaemia
SLE
Sydenham's chorea
Hyperthyroidism
Hypoparathyroidism

Choroidoretinitis
Toxoplasmosis
CMV (congenital)
Rubella (congenital)
Sarcoidosis
Diabetes mellitus

CK, ↑
Myocardial infarction, myocarditis
Muscle damage: surgery, trauma, burns, IM injections, rhabdomyolysis, rigorous
    exercise, seizures, haematoma, bowel ischaemia, dermatomyositis/
    polymyositis, defibrillation
Medications: statins, azathioprine, alcohol
Myxoedema
Muscular dystrophy

Clotting screen
PT: *See* Prothrombin time
APTT: *See* APTT
INR: *See* INR
TT: *See* Thrombin time
DIC: *See* Disseminated intravascular coagulation

Clubbing
Congenital
Acquired
Cardiovascular
Congenital cyanotic heart disease
Infective endocarditis
Atrial myxoma

Respiratory
Cancer: bronchial, mesothelioma
Fibrosis (e.g. cryptogenic fibrosing alveolitis)
Suppurative lung disease (abscess, bronchiectasis, empyema)
Cryptogenic organizing pneumonia (rare)

Gastrointestinal
Cirrhosis

Clubbing continued
Inflammatory bowel disease
GI lymphoma, malabsorption e.g. coeliac disease
Others: Thyroid acropachy (thyrotoxicosis), unilateral clubbing: axillary artery
    aneurysm, brachial AV malformations

Cold peripheries
Acute ischaemic limb (thromboembolism)
Raynaud's phenomenon (vasospasm)
Shock
Hypothyroidism
Drugs: β-blockers

Complement deficiency
Congenital e.g. C1 esterase (C1 inhibitor) deficiency (normal C3, ↓ C4)

Acquired
↓ C3 and C4:
    SLE, mixed cryoglobulinaemia
    Subacute bacterial endocarditis
    Serum sickness
    ↑ Loss/↓ synthesis: malnutrition, nephrotic syndrome, burns, liver failure
↓ C3
    Mesangiocapillary glomerulonephritis, partial lipodystrophy
    Gram −ve (endotoxic) shock
↑ C3 and/or C4
    Acute phase response

Consciousness, ↓
Hypoglycaemia
Hypoxia: cardiac arrest, shock (hypovolaemic, septic), respiratory failure
Vascular: intracranial haemorrhage/infarction
Infection: meningitis, encephalitis
Inflammation (demyelination)
Trauma (head injury)
Tumour (↑ intracranial pressure)
Toxic: drugs e.g. opiates, alcohol, anxiolytics, antidepressants
Metabolic: liver failure, renal failure, electrolyte (Na^+, K^+, Ca^{2+}, Mg^{2+})
    disturbances, endocrinopathies e.g. myxoedema coma, vitamin deficiencies
    (e.g. thiamine, B_{12}), hypothermia
Epilepsy
See also Blackouts

Constipation
Diet: low fibre, inadequate fluid intake
Drugs: opiates, anticholinergics (tricyclics, phenothiazines), iron
Immobility
Old age
Surgical/gastrointestinal:
    Anorectal disease (fissure, stricture, rectal prolapse)
    Intestinal obstruction (strictures, e.g. IBD, cancers, diverticulosis, pelvic mass,
        e.g. fibroids)
    Irritable bowel syndrome
    Post-operative

Endocrine: hypothyroidism, hypercalcaemia, hypokalaemia, porphyria, lead
 poisoning
Neurological/neuromuscular: autonomic neuropathy, spinal/pelvic nerve injury,
 scleroderma, Hirschsprung's disease, Chagas' disease

Corneal opacification
Corneal ulcer, keratitis
Acute angle closure glaucoma
Anterior uveitis (iritis)

Corneal ulcer
Bacterial infection (*Staphylococcus aureus/epidermidis, Pseudomonas,
 Streptococcus pneumoniae, Haemophilus*, coliforms)
Viral (herpes simplex, herpes zoster)
Fungal
Acanthamoeba
(Infections may follow corneal abrasion, contact lens wear or topical steroids)

Cottonwool spots
Diabetes (pre-proliferative retinopathy)
Hypertensive retinopathy
Retinal vein occlusion
HIV retinopathy
Haematological disorders: anaemia, leukaemia, hyperviscosity states
SLE, polyarteritis nodosa, dermatomyositis
Papilloedema

Cortisol, ↑
Stress, acute/chronic illness
Alcoholism
Cushing's syndrome (pituitary adenoma, adrenal adenoma/carcinoma, ectopic
 ACTH, e.g. bronchial carcinoids, ectopic CRH)
Depression
Exogenous glucocorticoids
↑ Cortisol-binding globulin (CBG): oestrogen, pregnancy

Cough
Upper respiratory tract infection
Pulmonary causes:
 All lung diseases e.g.
 Asthma, COPD, pulmonary emboli, infection (pneumonia, TB, fungal),
  bronchiectasis, malignancy, interstitial lung disease, sarcoidosis,
  pneumoconiosis
Other causes:
 Post-nasal drip
 Gastro-oesophageal reflux disease
 ACE inhibitors
 Heart failure
 Psychogenic

Crackles
Fine crackles
Pulmonary fibrosis (*See* Lung function tests, for the causes)
Pulmonary oedema

Crackles continued
Coarse crackles
Bronchiectasis
Consolidation (pneumonia)
COPD
(*Note*: crackles that disappear on coughing are not significant)

Cramp
Idiopathic
Flat feet, hypermobility syndrome, inappropriate leg positioning, prolonged
    sitting
Extracellular volume/salt depletion (diuretics, excessive sweating, fluid removal
    during haemodialysis)
Hypomagnesaemia
Hypokalaemia
Hypothyroidism
Drugs: β-agonists, Angiotensin II receptor blockers, cisplatin, vincristine
Muscle ischaemia, myopathy, motor neurone disease

Cranial nerve lesions
III
Vascular:
    Aneurysm: posterior communicating artery, basilar (in the brainstem), in the
        cavernous sinus
    Infarction in the brainstem
    Infarction in the nerve trunk ('medical' causes) diabetes, hypertension, SLE,
        polyarteritis nodosa, giant cell arteritis
    Thrombosis: in the cavernous sinus
Inflammation/infiltration of the basal meninges: TB, sarcoid, lymphoma,
    carcinoma, syphilis
Tumour: brainstem, cavernous sinus, superior orbital fissure/orbit tumour/
    granuloma
Tentorial herniation ('coning')
Brainstem CVA/demyelination/tumour
Cavernous sinus lesions (aneurysm, tumour, thrombosis)
Infective/carcinomatous meningitis
Orbital tumour
Nerve trunk infarction

IV
Head trauma

V
Sensory: trigeminal neuralgia, herpes zoster, nasopharyngeal carcinoma
Cerebellopontine angle tumour (acoustic neuroma, meningioma)
Brainstem CVA/tumour/demyelination
Cavernous sinus lesions (aneurysm, tumour, thrombosis)
Neoplastic infiltration of skull base
Petrositis (Gradenigo's syndrome)

VI
Damage to the nerve's blood supply (vasa nervosum): diabetes mellitus,
    hypertension
False localizing sign of ↑ intracranial pressure

Brainstem CVA/demyelination/tumour, Wernicke–Korsakoff syndrome
Cavernous sinus lesions
Cerebellopontine angle tumour
Infective/carcinomatous meningitis
Petrositis (Gradenigo's syndrome)
Orbital tumour

VII
See Facial nerve palsy

Multiple palsies
Trauma
Basal meningeal infiltration: carcinoma, TB, sarcoid, lymphoma,
    leukaemia
Brainstem lesions (CVA, tumour)
Guillain–Barré syndrome
Mononeuritis multiplex
Arnold–Chiari malformation
Paget's disease
See also Bulbar/pseudobulbar palsy and Jugular foramen syndrome for lower
    cranial nerve lesions.

Creatine kinase
See CK

Creatinine, plasma concentration
↑
↓ GFR (renal failure), high muscle mass, acute muscle damage (rhabdomyolysis)
Transient/minimal increase: after exercise, high meat meal
↓ Tubular secretion: trimethoprim, cimetidine

↓
↑ GFR (pregnancy)
Low muscle mass

Crepitations
See Crackles

CRP, ↑
Infection
Inflammation
Malignancy

Cryoglobulinaemia
Type I: Multiple myeloma, Waldenström's macroglobulinaemia
Type II: Chronic HCV infection, EBV, HBV
Type III: Inflammatory/autoimmune disorders (e.g. SLE, leukocytoclastic
    vasculitis), lymphoproliferative malignancies, HCV

CSF
↑ White cells
Predominantly lymphocytes
Infective meningitis: viral meningitis/meningoencephalitis, TB, fungal
    (Cryptococcal), listerial, syphilis

CSF continued

Inflammatory diseases, e.g. Behçet's disease, sarcoidosis, SLE, multiple sclerosis
Malignancy (meningeal infiltration): lymphoma, leukaemia, other tumours
Drugs: NSAIDs, trimethoprim

Predominantly neutrophils

Bacterial meningitis
Brain abscess eroding into the ventricles
Initial phase of viral meningitis (first 24–48 h)

↓ Glucose

Bacterial meningitis
TB meningitis
Fungal (cryptococcal) meningitis
Occasionally mumps meningitis & herpes encephalitis
Sarcoidosis, CNS vasculitides, carcinomatous meningitis

Normal cells, ↑ protein (cytoalbuminaemic dissociation)

Spinal block (tumour, epidural abscess)
Tumour
Guillain–Barré syndrome

Cyanosis

Central

↓ Oxygen transfer due to lung disease: fibrosing alveolitis, severe pneumonia, COPD, massive pulmonary embolism
R → L shunt (cyanotic congenital heart disease)
Methaemoglobinaemia, sulfhaemoglobinaemia
Acute: asthma, pneumothorax, inhaled foreign body, left ventricular failure

Peripheral

All causes of central cyanosis
Cold exposure
Raynaud's phenomenon
Arterial occlusion
↓ Cardiac output e.g. shock, left ventricular failure

D

Dactylitis
Psoriatic arthritis
Gonococcal arthritis
Sickle cell (bone marrow infarction)
Sarcoid (bone cysts)

Deafness
Conductive
Wax in the canal
Eardrum: perforation, cholesteatoma (chronic otitis media)
Otosclerosis, ossicular abnormality
Middle ear effusion (secondary to infection or malignancy)

Sensorineural
Infection: measles, mumps, meningitis, syphilis (rare)
Trauma: noise, head injury, surgery
Tumour: acoustic neuroma
Toxic: aminoglycosides, cytotoxic drugs, frusemide
Congenital: maternal rubella, eclampsia, perinatal hypoxia
Genetic: e.g. Alport syndrome, Waardenburg syndrome, DIDMOAD
Degenerative: presbyacusis
Others: Ménière's disease, Paget's disease of bone

Dehydration
↓ Fluid intake: severe illness, anorexia, malnutrition
Pyrexia/excess sweating
GI loss: diarrhoea, vomiting
Polyuria (e.g. diabetes mellitus, diabetes insipidus, hypercalcaemia)

Delirium (acute confusional state)
Hypoxia (respiratory/cardiac failure)
Hypoglycaemia
Toxic: alcohol (withdrawal, Wernicke's encephalopathy)
Drugs: opiates, anticholinergics, anxiolytics, anticonvulsants, corticosteroids,
    digoxin, dopaminergic agonists, recreational drugs
Metabolic: liver failure, renal failure, electrolyte imbalances (e.g. hyponatraemia,
    hypercalcaemia), endocrinopathies, nutritional deficiencies (B_{12}, nicotinic acid,
    thiamine)
Vascular: intracranial bleeding, infarction, venous sinus thrombosis
Infection: *Intracranial* (meningitis, encephalitis, abscess, cerebral malaria,
    neurocysticercosis), *Extracranial:* chest infection, urinary infection (esp.
    elderly), surgical wounds, IV lines
Inflammation: vasculitis
Trauma: head injury, subdural haematoma
Tumour: space-occupying lesions
Hypertensive encephalopathy
Epilepsy: status epilepticus, post-ictal states

Dementia
Alzheimer's disease
Vascular: multiple infarctions

Dementia continued

Infection: HIV, syphilis, Whipple's disease
Inflammation: vasculitis, SLE, sarcoid, multiple sclerosis
Trauma: head injury, subdural haemarrohage
Tumour: frontal tumours, posterior fossa (causing hydrocephalus), brain metastases, paraneoplastic
Toxic: alcohol, lead, barbiturates
Metabolic: myxoedema, vitamin B_{12} deficiency, hypoglycaemia (repeated)
Inherited: Wilson's disease, Huntington's chorea, some cerebellar ataxias
Degenerative: Parkinson's and other akinetic–rigid syndromes, Pick's disease, prion disease, Lewy body dementia

Desquamating rash

Toxic shock syndrome
Scarlet fever
Drug reaction
Kawasaki's disease

Diarrhoea

Infection: **Viral** (rotavirus, astrovirus, adenovirus, small round structured virus), Camylobacter, Salmonella, Shigella, E. coli, Yersinia enterocolitica, Staphylococcus aureus, Bacillus cereus, Clostridium botulinum, Clostridium perfringens, Clostridium difficile, Vibrio cholerae, Vibrio parahaemolyticus, **Parasites** (Cryptosporidia, Giardia, Entamoeba histolytica), **AIDS** (AIDS enteropathy, Cryptosporidia, Microsporidia, CMV)
Inflammatory bowel disease
Malabsorption: small intestine disease/resection
Medication: laxatives, antibiotics
Overflow diarrhoea: secondary to constipation
Endocrine: thyrotoxicosis, diabetes mellitus (autonomic neuropathy), VIPomas (Verner–Morrison syndrome)

Bloody diarrhoea

Infective colitis: Campylobacter, Haemorrhagic E. coli, Entamoeba histolytica, Salmonella, Shigella, (CMV in the immunocompromised)
Inflammatory bowel disease
Ischaemic colitis
Diverticulitis
Malignancy

Digital gangrene

Peripheral vascular disease, diabetes mellitus, Buerger's disease
Vasculitis, e.g. rheumatoid arthritis, polyarteritis nodosa, cryoglobulinaemia
Vasospasm: Raynaud's phenomenon
Emboli
Inadvertent intra-arterial injection in IV drug users
Subclavian artery compression (e.g. cervical rib)

Dimorphic blood film

Partially treat iron deficiency
Mixed iron and B_{12}/folate deficiency
Liver disease
Post-transfusion
Post-gastrectomy
Sideroblastic anaemia

Diplopia
Monocular
Originates from cornea or lens, e.g. cataract

Binocular
Cranial nerve palsies (III, IV, VI), See Cranial nerve lesions
Defective co-ordination between the nerves: internuclear ophthalmoplegia
Extra-ocular muscle disease (dysthyroid eye disease, myasthenia gravis, ocular myopathy, ocular myositis)
Orbital fracture

Disseminated intravascular coagulation
Infection: Gram −ve sepsis
Obstetric complications: missed abortion, severe pre-eclampsia, placental abruption, amniotic fluid emboli)
Malignancy: (AML: M3; adenocarcinoma)
Severe trauma
Surgery
Haemolytic transfusion reaction
Burns, snake bites, grafts

Dizziness
? Vertigo: See Vertigo
? Imbalance: See Ataxia
? Faintness: anaemia, blackouts (See Blackouts)

Dry eyes
↓ Tear production: ↓ Lipid layer (blepharitis), ↓ Aqueous layer (involvement of lacrimal glands: Sjögren's syndrome, rheumatoid arthritis, SLE, surgery, radiation), ↓ Mucin layer (↓ vitamin A, burns, circatricial pemphigoid)
Corneal epitheliopathy: trigeminal dysfunction, contact lens use
Drugs: antihistamines, antidepressants, β-blockers, contraceptive pills, diuretics
↓ Eyelid closure: facial nerve palsy, Graves' disease, prolonged reading

Dry mouth
Drugs: anticholinergics, antidepressants, antihistamines, diuretics, neuroleptics
Dehydration
Systemic disease: Sjögren's syndrome, sarcoidosis, amyloidosis, HIV, uncontrolled diabetes mellitus
Psychogenic: anxiety

Dullness at the lung base
Pleural effusion
Pleural thickening (old TB, empyema, mesothelioma)
Basal collapse
Raised hemidiaphragm (hepatomegaly, phrenic nerve palsy)

Dupuytren's contracture
Familial
↑ Frequency among alcoholics and diabetics

Dysarthria
Cerebellar disease: slurred, scanning speech
Bulbar palsy: nasal speech
Pseudobulbar palsy: slow, indistinct, effortful (spastic speech)
Extrapyramidal disease: soft, monotonous

Dysdiadochokinesis
See Cerebellar signs

Dysgeusia
Chronic nasal blockage
Old age
Facial nerve palsy
Drugs/toxins: metronidazole, ACE inhibitors, anti-thyroid drugs, Lithium,
    clarythromicin, heavy metals (e.g. lead poisoning)
Dental procedures
Rare:
Malignancy, bone marrow transplantation, GI (GORD, irritable bowel disease,
    cirrhosis)
Nutritional: Zn/B_{12} deficiency
Haemodialysis
HIV
Hypothyroidism
Depression
See also Ageusia

Dysmenorrhoea
Primary
No organic cause found

Secondary
Fibroids
Adenomyosis
Endometriosis
Pelvic inflammatory disease
Ovarian tumours

Dyspareunia
Superficial
Vulva: infection, dermatological disease, dysplasias
Vagina: infection, atrophic vaginitis (post-menopausal), dryness (Sjögren's
    syndrome, scleroderma), childbirth, episiotomy, surgery
Psychological

Deep
Endometriosis
Pelvic infection (chronic)
Pelvic mass
Irritable bowel syndrome

Dyspepsia
Oesophagus: gastro-oesophageal reflux, oesophagitis
Stomach/duodenum: peptic ulcer, hiatus hernia, gastritis, duodenitis, gastric
    cancer
Gall bladder: chronic cholecystitis
Non-ulcer dyspepsia

Dysphagia
Intraluminal
Foreign body

Intramural
Achalasia

Benign stricture: Oesophageal webs or rings
Cancer (oesophageal, gastric, pharyngeal)
Diffuse oesophageal spasm
Oesophagitis: infection, e.g. candidiasis, HSV, CMV, HIV or inflammation, e.g. GORD, corrosives, radiotherapy
Others: scleroderma, Chagas' disease

Extramural
Lung cancer
Lymphadenopathy
Retrosternal goitre
Pharyngeal pouch
Paraoesophageal hiatus hernia
Aortic aneurysm
Aberrant subclavian artery (dysphagia lusoria)
Atrial (left) enlargement

Neuromuscular
CVA
Guillain–Barré
Bulbar and pseudobulbar palsy
Myasthenia gravis
Inflammatory myositis
Motor neurone disease
Syringobulbia

Dysphasia
Broca's (expressive) dysphasia: lesions (e.g. CVA, tumour, trauma) affecting the infero-lateral frontal lobe (dominant)
Wernicke's (receptive) dysphasia: lesions (e.g. CVA, tumour, trauma) affecting the posterior superior temporal lobe (dominant)
Conduction dysphasia

Dyspnoea
See Breathlessness

Dystonia
Idiopathic
Drugs: antipsychotics (phenothiazines, chlorpromazine, haloperidol), antiemetics (metoclopramide), anticonvulsants
X-linked, e.g. Lesch–Nyhan syndrome
Autosomal dominant, e.g. spinocerebellar degenerations, Huntington's disease
Autosomal recessive, e.g. Wilson's disease
Mitochondrial disease

Dysuria
Urinary tract infection: cystitis, urethritis, acute pyelonephritis (uncommon cause of dysuria)
Urethritis: chlamydial, gonococcal, others: *Trichomonas vaginalis, Candida albicans*, Herpes simplex
Vaginitis: *Candida albicans, Trichomonas vaginalis*, bacterial vaginosis
Prostatitis
Interstitial cystitis
Female urethral syndrome

E

Ear ache
External ear
Trauma/subperichondral haematoma
Boil, furuncle
Otitis externa
Inclusion dermoid
Malignancy (e.g. squamous cell carcinoma, basal cell carcinoma)

Middle ear
Otitis media
Mastoiditis

Referred
Teeth
Tongue (tumour of the posterior third)
Tonsillitis, pharyngitis
Temporomandibular joint
Foreign body

Neurological
Herpes zoster
Glossopharyngeal neuralgia

ECG changes
Axis deviation (left and right): See Axis deviation
Bundle branch block (left and right): See Bundle branch block
Low voltage complexes: obesity, COPD, pleural effusion, myxoedema
P wave (absent and tall): See P wave
ST segment (elevation and depression): See ST segment
Tachycardia: See Tachycardia
U wave: See U wave

Emphysema, surgical
Trauma, surgery, chest drain insertion
Oesophageal injury
Positive pressure ventilation
Obstructive lung disease, e.g. asthma
Gas gangrene

Eosinophilia
See White cell count

Epistaxis
Trauma/irritation: nose picking, forceful blowing, foreign body,
    chronic intranasal drugs use (e.g. cocaine)
Nasal tumours
Anticoagulants, bleeding disorders
Hereditary haemorrhagic telangiectasia

Erythema multiforme
Idiopathic

Drugs: sulphonamides, penicillins, anticonvulsants
Infection: viral (HSV, EBV, orf), bacterial (*Mycoplasma pneumoniae*, chlamydiae), fungal (histoplasmosis, coccidiomycosis)
Inflammatory/connective tissue diseases: rheumatoid arthritis, SLA, sarcoidosis, PAN, Wegener's granulomatosis
Malignancy (lymphoma, leukaemia, myeloma), radiation

Erythema nodosum

Infection: **Bacterial** (*Streptococcus, Chlamydia*, TB, *Yersinia, Rickettsia*, leprosy, leptospirosis), **Viral** (EBV), **Fungal** (histoplasmosis, coccidiomycosis, blastomycosis), **Protozoal** (toxoplasmosis)
Inflammation: inflammatory bowel disease, sarcoidosis, Behçet's disease
Malignancy: lymphoma, leukaemia
Drugs: sulphonamides, penicillin, oral contraception, salicylates, dapsone
Pregnancy

ESR

↑
Infection
Inflammatory/connective tissue diseases
Malignancy
Metabolic, e.g. phaeochromocytoma

↑ESR, normal CRP

SLE
Ulcerative colitis
Myeloma
Recovery from an infection: when CRP has normalized but ESR is still high (has a longer half-life)

Exophthalmos

See Proptosis

Eyelids, swollen

Allergy (contact with cosmetics, chemicals, animals, plants)
Blepharitis (may be associated with rosacea, eczema, psoriasis)
Chalazion, stye, spread of infection from a local lesion e.g. a squeezed comedo
Dacryocytitis

More serious causes

Orbital cellulitis
Herpes zoster ophthalmicus
Herpes simplex

Eye pain

See Painful red eye
Pain on eye movement
   Optic neuritis
   Orbital myositis

F

Facial nerve palsy
Unilateral
Bell's palsy (idiopathic)
Trauma or surgery of the face
Tumours: brainstem, cerebellopontine angle (acoustic neuroma), meningeal
    infiltration, parotid gland
Vascular: brainstem infarction
Infection (petrous bone): middle ear infection or herpes zoster
Inflammation: sarcoidosis (meningeal inflammation), multiple sclerosis
    (demyelination in brainstem)

Bilateral
Congenital facial diplegia
Guillain–Barré syndrome
Sarcoidosis
Motor nurone disease
Myasthenia gravis
Muscular dystrophy
Infections: Lyme disease, HIV

Facial pain
Neurological
Giant cell arteritis
Trigeminal neuralgia
Glossopharyngeal neuralgia
Migrainous neuralgia and migraine
Postherpetic neuralgia

Local causes
Post-traumatic
Sinusitis
Orbital and ocular disease, optic neuritis, retro-orbital disease (e.g. posterior
    communicating artery aneurysm)
Dental/oral disease
Temporomandibular joint dysfunction
Ear and parotid disease
Nasopharyngeal tumours
Referred cardiac pain
Atypical facial pain

Facial swelling
Periorbital oedema
Infection: orbital/periorbital cellulitis, trichinosis (rare)
Allergy to insect bites/drugs (including anaphylaxis), C1 inhibitor deficiency
Hypo/hyperthyroidism
Nephrotic syndrome, hypoalbuminaemia
Carotico-cavernous fistula, cavernous sinus thrombosis
Dermatomyositis

Parotid enlargement
See Parotid enlargement

Other causes of facial swelling/enlargement
Dental/sinus infection
Trauma, burns
Subcutaneous emphysema
SVC thrombosis
Cushing's syndrome, obesity

Faecal incontinence
Diarrhoea (*See* Diarrhoea)
Overflow (faecal impaction, rectal neoplasm)
Pelvic floor abnormality: accidental injury, e.g. pelvic fracture, anorectal surgery, obstetric-traumatic childbirth, rectal prolapse
Neurological: epilepsy, spinal cord compression, stroke, multiple sclerosis, trauma and tumours (brain, spinal cord, cauda equina), peripheral neuropathy (e.g. diabetes), dementia, Parkinson's disease
Congenital: meningomyelocele, anorectal anomalies

Fasciculations
Motor neurone disease
Motor root compression
Polyneuropathy
Primary myopathy
Thyrotoxicosis

Fatigue
Anaemia
Endocrine/metabolic: diabetes mellitus, hypo/hyperthyroidism, Addison's disease, uraemia
Heart failure
Infection
Inflammatory/connective tissue diseases
Malignancy
Drugs, e.g. β-blockers
Depression
Chronic fatigue syndrome

Ferritin ($\uparrow$&$\downarrow$)
$\uparrow$
Acute phase response: infection, inflammation, malignancy
Haemochromatosis
Repeated transfusions in thalassaemia, iron therapy
Still's disease
Sideroblastic anaemia
Anaemia of chronic disease, chronic haemolysis

$\downarrow$
Iron deficiency

Fever in traveller
Hepatitis A
Malaria
Typhoid
Leptospirosis
Dengue
Haemorrhagic fevers

Fever in traveller continued
Longer incubation
Malaria
Typhoid
TB
Brucellosis
Leishmaniasis
Amoebic abscess

Fever of unknown origin
See Pyrexia of unknown origin

Finger pain
Trauma: fracture, subungal haematocoma
Arthritis: e.g. rheumatoid arthritis, gout
Infection: paronychia, tendon sheath infection, pulp space infection
Ischaemia: vasospasm (Raynaud's phenomenon), vasculitis, peripheral vascular disease, emboli
Carpal tunnel syndrome
Referred: cervical spondylosis
Other: scleroderma, tumours (bone tumour, glomus tumour)

Flaccid paraparesis
Polyneuropathies (*See* Polyneuropathy)
Myopathies
Tabes dorsalis

Flatulence
See under Belching, bloating and flatulence

Floaters
Vitreous degeneration/detachment
Vitreous haemorrhage
Posterior uveitis (e.g. toxoplasmosis, sarcoidosis)

Flushing, facial
Physiological: heat, exertion, emotion
Menopause
Phaeochromocytoma
Carcinoid syndrome
Drugs: alcohol (particularly with chlorpropamide), testosterone, nitrites
Rosacea

Folate deficiency
↑ Demand: pregnancy/lactation, malignancy, chronic inflammation, chronic haemolytic anaemia, haemodialysis
↓ Absorption: jejunal disease, e.g. coeliac disease, tropical sprue, Whipple's disease, small intestinal resection
↓ Intake: alcoholics, elderly, anorexia
Drugs: phenytoin, trimethoprim, sulfasalazine

Foot drop
Neurological
Common peroneal nerve lesion: mononeuritis multiplex, e.g. diabetes mellitus (*See* Mononeuritis multiplex)

L5 root lesion (radiculopathy), e.g. inter-vertebral disc prolapse
Rarer: motor neuron disease, multiple sclerosis, stroke
Muscular
Injury to the dorsiflexors, compartment syndrome

Foot pain
Deformities (e.g. flat feet), strain (muscular, ligamentous strain)
Skin: cellulitis, warts, corns, callosities
Bone: fracture (calcaneal fracture, metatarsal fracture), osteomyelitis,
    osteochondritis:, e.g. metatarsal head (Freiberg's disease) and navicular
    (Köhler's disease), tumours
Joints: septic arthritis, gout, rheumatoid arthritis, osteoarthritis (see
    Monoarthralgia and Polyarthralgia)
Periarticular: plantar fasciitis, tendonitis (e.g. Achilles tendon, peroneal tendon,
    tibialis posterior), bursitis (e.g. retro and infracalcaneal, interMTP)
Vascular: ischaemia, ulcers (see Digital gangrene)
Neurological: L4/L5/S1 root pain, Morton's metatarsalgia (plantar nerve
    neuroma), tarsal tunnel syndrome

Frequency (urinary), nocturia
Polyuria (See Polyuria)
Frequent passage of small amounts of urine: UTI, bladder (stone, tumour,
    compression by pelvic mass), prostate enlargement (BPH, cancer), genuine
    stress incontinence, detrusor instability, sensory urgency

Frontal bossing
Acromegaly
Paget's disease of the bone
Rickets
Thalassaemia
Hydrocephalus
Rarer causes: Gorlin's syndrome, achondroplasia

G

Gait
Antalgic gait due to pain
Leg length discrepancies
Waddling: *See* Proximal myopathy
Spastic, scissoring: *See* Spastic paraparesis
Wide-base: *See* Ataxia
Festinant, shuffling gait: Parkinson's disease
Steppage gate: peroneal nerve palsy, Charcot–Marie–Tooth disease, old polio, heavy metal poisoning, e.g. lead
Apraxic gaits: frontal lobe lesions

Galactorrhoea
See Hyperprolactinaemia

Gastrointestinal bleeding, upper and lower
Upper GI bleeding (haematemesis)
Peptic ulcer (gastric/duodenal)
Gastritis/gastric erosions, duodenitis, oesophagitis
Gastro-oesophageal varices
Mallory–Weiss tear
Medications: NSAIDs, anticoagulants, steroids, thrombolytics
Oesophageal/gastric cancer

Rare
Bleeding disorders (thrombocytopenia, haemophilia), hereditary haemorrhagic telangiectasia, Dieulafoy gastric vascular abnormality, aortoduodenal fistulae, angiodysplasia, leiomyoma, Meckel's diverticulum, pseudoxanthoma elasticum

Lower GI bleeding
Anal: haemorrhoids, fissure
Angiodysplasia
Bowel cancer, polyps
Colitis: inflammatory (ulcerative colitis), infective, ischaemic, radiation
Diverticulae (colonic)
Excessive upper GI bleeding
Other: bleeding disorders, aortoenteric fistula, Meckel's diverticulum, solitary rectal ulcer

Gaze palsy
Horizontal
Ipsilateral pontine (pontine paramedian reticular formation) or Contralateral frontal lobe lesions:
Vascular (infarction/haemorrhage, vascular malformations), tumour, demyelination, infection

Vertical
Superior midbrain lesions:
Vascular (infarction/haemorrhage, vascular malformations), tumours (pinealoma/metastatic), demyelination, infection, metabolic (e.g. Niemann–Pick disease,

Gaucher's disease, abetalipoproteinemia), neurodegenerative (Steele–Richardson syndrome: associated with extrapyramidal dysfunction)

Note: In Parinaud's syndrome, paralysis of vertical gaze is associated with large pupils and light–near dissociation.

Genital discharge (males)
Physiological
Sexual arousal, smegma, crystalluria, prostatorrhoea

Pathological
Urethra: gonorrhoea, chlamydia, non-specific infection, trichmoniasis, herpes, 2° to intra-urethral lesions, 2° to prostatitis/upper urinary traction infection/lesion
Prepuce/glans: candidiasis, herpes, balanoposthitis

Genital rash
See Ulcers, genital

Genital ulcers
See Ulcers, genital

Gingival hypertrophy
Familial
Drugs: ciclosporin, phenytoin, Ca channel antagonists (nifedipine, diltiazem), OCP
Acute leukaemia
Tuberous sclerosis
Pregnancy

Glossitis
Iron deficiency
Deficiency of folate, B_{12}, niacin (B_3), thiamine (B_1), riboflavin, Zn
Candidiasis
Syphilis (rare)

γ–glutamyl transpeptidase (Y-GT, GGT)
Liver disease: cholestasis (*See* under Jaundice), alcohol-induced damage

Glycosuria
Diabetes (1° and 2°: see Hyperglycaemia)
Pregnancy
Chronic renal failure
Renal tubular dysfunction/damage (e.g. multiple myeloma, heavy metals, Wilson's disease)

Goitre
Simple goitre (euthyroid): puberty, pregnancy
Hyperthyroidism: Graves' disease, toxic adenoma, toxic multinodular goitre with one palpable nodule, thyroiditis
Hypothyroidism: Hashimoto's disease
Lithium, antithyroid drugs, iodine deficiency/excess, dyshormogenesis
Thyroid cyst
Thyroid carcinoma: papillary, follicular, anaplastic, medullary, lymphoma

γ-GT, ↑
See γ–glutamyl transpeptidase

Groin pain
See Abdominal pain

Gynaecomastia

Physiological: puberty, elderly

Pseudogynaecomastia: e.g. in obese men

Drugs: spirinolactone, cimetidine, cyproterone acetate, chlorpromazine, oestrogens, digoxin, drugs of abuse (heroin, marijuana)

Chronic liver disease

Chronic renal failure

Hypogonadism

Hyperthyroidism

Tumours: ectopic hCG (e.g. hepatoma and lung), oestrogen-producing (e.g. testicular)

Unilateral

Breast carcinoma

Lipoma, lymphangioma, neurofibroma, haematoma, dermoid cyst

H

Haematemesis
See Gastrointestinal bleeding

Haemarthrosis
Trauma: iatrogenic, post-operative, fracture, meniscus tear, ligamentous injury (e.g. anterior cruciate)
Haematological: Clotting disorders, sickle cell disease, drugs
Infection: Septic arthritis, TB
Vascular: haemangioma, arteriovenous malformation, aneurysm
Neurological: Charcot's joint
Joint diseases: Osteoarthritis, gout, pseudogout
Scurvy
Tumour: pigmented villonodular synovitis

Haematuria
Kidney, bladder, ureter or urethra
Trauma
Infection: UTI, rarely TB, schistosomiasis
Stones
Tumours
Other causes: glomerulonephritis, IgA nephropathy, interstitial nephritis, cystic renal disease, emboli, renal vein thrombosis, vascular malformation, drugs, e.g. cyclophosphamide, excessive exercise
Prostate: benign prostatic hyperplasia, prostate cancer, prostatitis
General: haematological disorders (haemophilia, thrombocytopenia, sickle cell disease, leukaemia), anticoagulants

Other causes of urine discoloration
Food: beetroot
Drugs (senna, rifamipcin)
Haemoglobinuria/myoglobinuria
Porphyria (acute intermittent)

Haemoglobin
↓
See Anaemia

↑
See Polycythaemia

Haemoptysis
Lung: infection (TB, pneumonia, abscess, bronchitis, bronchiectasis fungi, parasites), pulmonary embolism, malignancy, vasculitis (e.g. Wegener's granulomatosis, Goodpasture's disease), trauma, foreign body
Heart: mitral stenosis
General bleeding diathesis
Rarer causes: arteriovenous malformation, amyloidosis, sarcoidosis
Note: Nasal/upper respiratory tract and GI bleeding may be confused with haemoptysis

Hair loss
See Alopecia

Halitosis
Mouth: Poor dental hygiene, dental plaque, gingivitis, oropharyngeal
  malignancy
Nasopharynx: Atrophic rhinitis, chronic sinusitis and post-nasal drip, chronic
  tonsillitis, pharyngeal pouch
GI: achalasia, oesophageal stricture, GORD
Lung: infections, bronchiectasis

Hallucination
Psychiatric
Schizophrenia/schizoaffective disorder
Mania with psychosis
Severe depression with psychosis
Dementia
Delirium
Puerperal psychosis
Alcoholic hallucinosis

Organic
Cerebrovascular (stroke), infection, toxic/metabolic (e.g. alcohol, hallucinogens,
  e.g. LSD), drug-induced psychosis (e.g. amphetamine, cocaine)
Sensory organ disease, e.g. retinal ischaemia/optic nerve lesions
Seizures

Hand pain
See Finger pain

Hands, enlarged
Acromegaly
Amyloidosis
Hypothyroidism
Obesity
Manual work

Headache
Acute/subacute causes (likely to present in A&E)
Head injury
Meningitis/encephalitis
Subarachnoid haemorrhage, intracranial haemorrhage, cerebral venous
  thrombosis
Carotid/vertebral artery dissection
Acute angle closure glaucoma
Giant cell arteritis
Pituitary apoplexy
Other causes: ↑ ↑ BP, drugs (e.g. GTN, Ca channel antagonists), infections
  (bacterial, viral illnesses etc.), electrolyte imbalances (e.g. hyponatraemia),
  hyperviscosity syndromes (e.g. polycythaemia)

Chronic/recurrent
↑ Intracranial pressure (e.g. space occupying lesion, e.g. tumour/abscess,
  hydrocephalus, benign intracranial hypertension) and ↓ intracranial pressure
  (e.g. post lumbar puncture)

Migraine
Migrainous neuralgia
Tension headache, rebound headache (on stopping analgesics)
Sinusitis
Other causes: cervicogenic (referred from cervical spondylosis), hypnic
    headache, meningeal infiltration (e.g. malignancy, sarcoidosis), refractive
    errors, Paget's disease of bone, acromegaly, antiphospholipid syndrome
See also Facial pain

Heart sounds
First (S1)
Loud (↑ intensity)
Mitral stenosis, atrial myxoma
Tachycardia, hyperdynamic circulation (e.g. fever, exercise)
↓ PR interval (pre-excitation syndromes)

Soft (↓ intensity)
Mitral regurgitation
Artic regurgitation
Long PR interval
LBBB
Severe heart failure

Variable intensity
Atrial fibrillation
AV block
Nodal or ventricular tachycardia

Second (S2)
Loud
Systemic hypertension, tachycardia (↑ a_2)
Pulmonary hypertension (↑ p_2)

Soft
Aortic stenosis (↓ a_2)
Pulmonary stenosis (↓ p_2)

Third (S3)
Normal in those < 35 years
Ventricular failure
Mitral regurgitation, tricuspid regurgitation, VSD
Constrictive pericarditis, restrictive cardiomyopathy

Fourth (S4)
Aortic stenosis
Hypertensive heart disease
Hypertrophic cardiomyopathy
Myocardial infarction
Pulmonary stenosis

Splitting of S2
Wide
Delayed activation of right ventricle
RBBB, left ventricular pacing, left ventricular preexcitation (Wolff–
    Parkinson–White syndrome)

Heart sounds continued

Prolonged right ventricular ejection time
Pulmonary stenosis, pulmonary hypertension

↓ Left ventricular ejection time
Mitral regurgitation, VSD

Wide fixed splitting
ASD

Reversed splitting
Delayed activation of left ventricle
LBBB, right ventricular pacing, right ventricular preexcitation

Prolonged left ventricular ejection time
Aortic stenosis, HOCM, hypertension, PDA

Single S2
Apparent: obesity, COPD, pericardial effusion
Absent a_2: severe aortic stenosis, severe aortic regurgitation
Absent p_2: absent pulmonary valve, pulmonary atresia, pulmonary stenosis,
   tetralogy of Fallot
Fusion of a_2 and p_2: Eisenmenger's syndrome

↓ Heart sounds
↓ Conduction of sounds: obesity, COPD, pericardial effusion

Heart murmurs
See Murmurs

Heinz bodies (denatured Hb)
G6PD deficiency
Haemolytic anaemias
Splenectomy

Hemianopia
Bitemporal
Superior temporal quadrants involved first
Pituitary adenoma, meningioma, carotid aneurysm
Nasopharyngeal carcinoma
Sphenoid sinus mucocele

Inferior temporal quadrants involved first
Craniopharyngioma
Third ventricular tumour

Homonymous
Involvement of:
Optic tract or
Optic radiation (in parietal or temporal lobes) or
Occipital cortex by: CVA (sudden): stroke/transient ischaemic attack (TIA)
Masses: gliomas, metastasis, abscess

Hemiparesis, hemiplegia

Vascular: CVA (infarction, haemorrhage, TIA)
Infection: brain abscess from local (e.g. middle ear, sinuses) or distant (e.g. lung) infections
Inflammation: multiple sclerosis, cerebral vasculitis
Trauma: extradural or subdural haemorrhage (a history of trauma may not be apparent in the latter)
Tumour
Metabolic: hypoglycaemia can cause transient hemiplegia
Other causes of transient hemiplegia/paresis: epileptic seizures (Todd's paralysis), migraine

Hepatomegaly

Cancer: (2° deposits, hepatoma, liver cell adenoma)
Cirrhosis (early) usually alcoholic, primary biliary cirrhosis
Congestive cardiac failure
Budd–Chiari (hepatic vein thrombosis)
Polycystic liver disease
Infection: hepatitis A, B, C, EBV, CMV, toxoplasmosis, leptospirosis, abscess (amoebic, pyogenic), hydatid cyst
Infiltration: fatty infiltration (alcohol), haemochromatosis, amyloidosis, sarcoidosis, lymphoproliferative diseases
'Apparent hepatomegaly': lowered diaphragm (e.g. in COPD) or Reidle's lobe (an extension of the right lobe)
Also see Hepatosplenomegaly

Hepatosplenomegaly

Myeloproliferative disorders*
Lymphoproliferative disorders**
Portal hypertension (See Portal hypertension)
Megaloblastic anaemia (e.g. pernicious anaemia)
Infection: hepatitis B or C, EBV, CMV, leptospirosis, toxoplasmosis, tuberculosis, brucellosis
    Worldwide: malaria, schistosomiasis, leishmaniasis
Other: amyloidosis, storage disorders, e.g. Gaucher's disease, infantile polycystic disease

*Chronic myeloid leukaemia, myelofibrosis, polycythaemia rubra vera, essential thrombocythaemia
**Lymphoma, CLL, myeloma, Waldenström's macroglobulinaemia, ALL, hairy cell leukaemia

Hiccups
Benign

Gastric distension: over eating, carbonated beverages, aerophagia, gastric insufflation during endoscopy
Excessive alcohol ingestion and tobacco use; sudden changes in ambient or GI temperature, sudden excitement

Phrenic nerve irritation

Neck masses (e.g. goitres), mediastinal masses
Diaphragmatic abnormalities:, e.g. gastro-oesophageal reflux, hiatus hernia, intra-operative manipulation
Subdiaphragmatic:, e.g. subphrenic abscess

Hiccups continued
Vagus nerve irritation
Irritation of the recurrent laryngeal nerve by pharyngitis, laryngitis, tumours of
the neck
Irritation of the auricular branch of the vagus by foreign bodies touching the
tympanic membrane

Toxic/metabolic
Uraemia, alcohol intoxication, general anaesthetic

CNS disorders
Vascular, infective or structural lesions releasing the normal inhibition of the
hiccup reflex

Psychogenic
Anxiety, malingering

Hirsutism
Familial, racial (common in some Mediterranean and Indian subcontinent
populations)
Ovaries: PCOS, androgen-secreting ovarian tumours (e.g. arrhenoblastoma which
is a Sertoli–Leydig cell tumour)
Adrenals: Congenital adrenal hyperplasia, androgen-secreting adrenal tumours,
Cushing's syndrome
Drugs: ciclosporin, androgens, minoxidil, phenytoin
Target organ hypersensitivity

Hoarse voice
Laryngitis: *Acute* (associated with viral upper respiratory tract infection, acute
vocal strain), *Chronic* (associated with chronic vocal cord strain, alcohol,
smoking, GORD, postnasal drip, chemical fumes)
Recurrent laryngeal nerve injury: tumours (base of skull, neck, e.g. thyroid,
mediastinum, e.g. lung cancer), surgery (thyroid, parathyroid, carotid
endarterectomy)
Singer's nodules
Laryngeal trauma (e.g. intubation)
Laryngeal carcinoma
Hypothyroidism
Hysterical aphonia

Homocysteine, ↑
Genetic: Cystathionine β-synthetase deficiency, MTHFR polymorphism
Vitamin deficiency: B_6, B_{12}, folate
Drugs: methotrexate, theophylline, phenytoin
Disease: hypothyroidism, renal failure, breast/ovarian cancer
Lifestyle: aging, smoking, ↑↑ coffee consumption

Horner's syndrome
Brain stem/cervical spinal cord: tumour (glioma), infarction,
syringomyelia/bulbia
T1 root: brachial plexus lesion, neurofibromatosis
Cervical sympathetic chain: Pancoast tumour (lung apex)
Internal carotid artery: dissection, occlusion

Howell–Jolly bodies
Post-splenectomy
Hyposplenism: sickle cell disease, coeliac disease/dermatitis herpetiformis,
    ulcerative colitis, tropical sprue, amyloidosis, essential thrombocythaemia
Iron deficiency
Megaloblastic anaemia
Leukaemia

Hyperaldosteronism
$1°$ hyperaldosteronism: adenoma (Conn's syndrome), bilateral adrenal
    hyperplasia, glucocorticoid-remediable aldosteronism
$2°$ hyperaldosteronism: ↑ Renin: renin-secreting tumour, renal artery stenosis,
    cirrhosis, cardiac failure, diuretics, Bartter's syndrome

Hyperbilirubinaemia
Unconjugated: haemolysis (See Anaemia, haemolytic), ineffective erythropoiesis,
    ↓ glucuronidation (Gilbert's syndrome, Crigler–Najjar syndrome)
Conjugated: See Jaundice, hepatocellular and obstructive

Hypercalcaemia
Hyperparathyroidism: primary and tertiary
Malignancy: multiple myeloma, bone metastasis: (prostate, kidney, thyroid,
    breast, lung), bronchial squamous cell carcinoma, lymphoma
Excess vitamin D: self-administered, sarcoid, TB
Immobility

Other causes
↑ Ca^{2+} intake ('milk alkali syndrome')
Drugs: Lithium, thiazides
Endocrine diseases: hyperthyroidism, phaeochromocytoma, acromegaly,
    Addison's disease
Familial hypocalciuric hypercalcaemia
Hypercalcaemia can also occur in diuretic phase of acute renal failure

Hypercalciuria
Hypercalcaemia (see above)
Idiopathic hypercalciuria
↑ Ca^{2+} intake
Renal tubular acidosis
X-linked hypercalciuria (Dent's disease)

Hypergammaglobulinaemia
Polyclonal
Chronic liver disease, primary biliary cirrhosis, autoimune hepatitis
Chronic inflammatory/connective tissue disease (e.g. Sjögren's syndrome,
    sarcoidosis, SLE, rheumatoid arthritis, dermatomyositis), inflammatory bowel
    disease
Chronic infection (e.g. bronchiectasis), TB, brucellosis, leishmaniasis, leprosy, HIV
    infection

Monoclonal
See Paraproteinaemia

Hyperglycaemia
Stress, e.g. acute/severe illness
Steroids

Diabetes
Primary (type 1 & 2)
Secondary:
Steroids
Endocrine: Cushing's syndrome, acromegaly, phaeochromocytomas, glucagonomas, somatostatinomas
Pancreatectomy, chronic pancreatitis, haemochromatosis

Hyperhidrosis
Endocrine: thyrotoxicosis, acromegaly, phaeochromocytoma
Chronic infection: TB, brucellosis
Malignancy: lymphoma
Medications: opiates, drugs with cholinergic properties, sympathomimetics
Acute: any acute febrile illness, myocardial infarction, hypoglycaemia, hypotension
Also See Night sweats

Hyperkalaemia
Released from cells: acidosis, rhabdomyolysis, suxamethonium
Renal failure
Renal tubular acidosis type 4
ACE inhibitors
Addison's disease
Amiloride and other potassium-sparing diuretics
↑↑ Intake
Pseudohyperkalaemia: haemolysis, leucocytosis, thrombocytosis

Hyperkeratosis (palmoplantar)
Friction (e.g. walking barefoot)
Congenital (tylosis, an autosomal dominant condition)
Keratoderma blenorrhagica (Reiter's syndrome)
Psoriasis
2° syphilis
Toxic/metabolic: drug reaction, arsenic, vitamin A deficiency
Malignancy: gastric adenocarcinoma, bronchial carcinoma

Hyperlipidaemia (2°)
Diabetes (poorly controlled)
Drugs: alcohol, OCP, steroids, thiazides
Myxoedema
Nephrotic syndrome, renal impairment
Obesity
Obstructive jaundice

Hypernatraemia
Dehydration:
↓ Fluid intake: elderly, confused or unconscious
↑ Fluid loss GI: diarrhoea vomiting
　　Renal: diabetes insipidus, osmotic diuresis (e.g. hyperglycaemia, hypercalcaemia)
　　Skin: excessive sweating
　　Hyperosmolar non-ketotic coma

Excess Na$^+$ administration (e.g. sodium bicarbonate)
Excess mineralocortcoids: hyperaldosteronism

Hyperparathyroidism
1° hyperparathyroidism
Parathyroid adenoma or hyperplasia (may be associated with MEN syndromes)
and rarely carcinoma

2° hyperparathyroidism?
↓ Calcium (e.g. due to vitamin D deficiency or resistance or chronic renal failure)

3° hyperparathyroidism
Autonomous parathyroid hyperplasia secondary to long-standing 2°
hyperparathyroidism

Hyperphosphataemia
Renal failure
Hypo & Pseudohypoparathyroidism (PTH: Phosphate Trashing Hormone!)
Rhabdomyolysis
Tumour lysis syndrome
Acromegaly
Excessive phosphate intake/administration
Vitamin D intoxication

Hyperpigmentation
Drugs: amiodarone, busulfan, chlorpromazine, phenothiazines
Radiation
Endocrine: Addison's disease, Nelson's syndrome, ectopic ACTH,
pregnancy
Liver disease: haemochromatosis, primary biliary cirrhosis
Photosensitive rashes *See* Photodistributed rash
Post-inflammatory, e.g. after erythroderma
Others: chronic renal failure, chronic wasting (TB, carcinoma), disseminated
malignant melanomatosis

Hyperprolactinaemia
Physiological: pregnancy, lactation, stress
Prolactinoma, rarely ectopic prolactin (lung, kidney tumours)
↓ Dopamine transport to the anterior pituitary: pituitary tumour compressing
pituitary stalk (pseudoprolactinoma affect)
Drugs:
Depletion of central dopamine stores: reserpine, methyldopa
Dopamine receptor blockers: (chlorpromazine, haloperidol, sulpiride,
metoclopramide, domperidone)
↑ TRH secretion stimulates prolactin release (1° hypothyroidism)
Oestrogens: HRT/OCP, PCOS (oestrogen stimulates lactotrophs)
Chest wall injury (stimulation of the reflex pathway normally activated by
suckling in lactating women)
Others: liver failure, ↓ dopamine synthesis/release from the hypothalamus
(tumour, inflammation, arteriovenous malformations)

Hyperproteinaemia
Haemoconcentration: dehydration, prolonged application of tourniquet
Hypergammaglobulinaemia: *See* Hypergammaglobulinaemia

Hypertension
Essential (idiopathic)
Renal disease: chronic glomerulonephritis, chronic pyelonephritis, cystic kidney disease, renal carcinoma
Drugs: oestrogen-containing OCPs, steroids
Endocrine disease: Cushing's syndrome, Conn's disease, phaeochromocytomas, acromegaly, primary hyperparathyroidism
Vascular: coarctation of aorta, renal artery stenosis
Pre-eclampsia

Hyperthyroidism
Graves' disease
Toxic multinodular goitre
Toxic adenoma
Thyroiditis (subacute/viral, post-partum)
Gestational thyrotoxicosis ($\uparrow$ hCG)

Rarer causes
Secondary hyperthyroidism (TSH)
Follicular carcinoma of thyroid
Choreocarcinoma
Struma ovarii
Drugs: amiodarone, surreptitious thyroxine consumption (thyroiditis factitia)
TSH-receptor mutations, McCune–Albright syndrome

Hypertrichosis
Local
Lichen simplex
Melanocytic naevi
Spina bifida

Generalized
Anorexia nervosa
Malnutrition
Medication (minoxidil, ciclosporin, phenytoin),
Malignancy
Porphyria cutanea tarda

Hyperuricaemia
$\downarrow$ Renal excretion
Idiopathic
Drugs: **c**iclosporin, **a**spirin (low-dose), **n**icotinic acid, **t**hiazides, **l**oop diuretics, **e**thambutol, **a**lcohol, **p**yrizinamide)
Chronic renal disease, e.g. in diabetes mellitus, hypertension

$\uparrow$ Intake/production
$\uparrow$ Dietary intake
$\uparrow$ Synthesis: Lesch–Nyhan syndrome (HGPRT deficiency)
$\uparrow$ Nucleic acid (purine) turnover: lymphoma, leukaemia, polycythaemia vera, psoriasis

Hypoalbuminaemia
$\downarrow$ Synthesis
Acute phase reaction

Liver disease
Malnutrition

↑ Loss
Nephrotic syndrome
Protein-losing enteropathy (coeliac disease, IBD, sprue, Whipple's disease,
    intestinal lymphoma, intestinal lymphangiectasia)
Burns
Bullous skin lesions

Haemodilution
Sample from IV infusion arm, pregnancy

Rare
Familial idiopathic dysproteinaemia

Hypocalcaemia
Hypoparathyroidism
    Congenital (DiGeorge's syndrome)
    Autoimmune
    Surgical (after thyroidectomy or parathyroidectomy)
    Pseudohypoparathyroidism (resistance to PTH)
    ↓ Mg^{2+}, Fe^{2+} overload, ↑ Cu^{2+} (Wilson's disease)
Vitamin D deficiency
    ↓ Dietary intake/malabsorption
    Lack of sunlight
    Liver disease
    Anticonvulsants (e.g. phenytoin)
    Renal failure
    Vitamin D resistance
↑ Phosphate: chronic renal failure, phosphate therapy
Pancreatitis (acute)
Respiratory alkalosis
Hypoalbuminaemia
Others
    Artifact (collecting blood into an EDTA tube)
    Iatrogenic: bisphosphonates, calcitonin, citrated blood (massive transfusion)

Hypochromia
Iron deficiency anaemia
Thalassaemia
Sideroblastic anaemia

Hypogammaglobulinaemia
Congenital
X-linked, or as part of a combined immunodeficiency state

Acquired
Myeloma
Lymphoma
Leukaemia (CLL)
Nephrotic syndrome, malnutrition, malabsorption, protein-losing enteropathy
Marrow hypoplasia, myeloclerosis
Uraemia, steroids, severe infections

Hypoglycaemia

Excess insulin (or diabetics not having a snack after insulin injection), sulphonylureas, salicylate, pentamidine, quinine
Insulinomas, hepatomas, sarcomas
Alcohol
Addison's disease
Renal failure
Liver failure
Malaria
Post-gastrectomy

Hypogonadism

Female

1° hypogonadism (hypergonadotrophic)

Gonadal dysgensis

The genotype may be XO (Turner's syndrome), XX, XY (with disruption of the *SRY* gene on Y chromosome or the downstream pathway), XO/XY or XO/XX (mosaicism)

Gonadal damage

Infection (e.g. mumps)
Autoimmune
Surgery (pelvic)
Radiation
Chemotherapy, e.g. cyclophosphamide

Genetic mutations

LH/FSH beta subunit, LH receptor, FSH receptor, enzymes involved in oestrogen synthesis (e.g. 17-hydroxylase deficiency), galactosaemia

2° hypogonadism (hypogonadotrophic)

Hypopituitarism

Pituitary tumour/surgery/radiation, infiltrations (e.g. lymphoma, sarcoidosis, Langerhans cell histiocytosis, lymphocytic hypophysitis)
Functional/hypothalamic, e.g. strenuous exercise, weight loss
Congenital GnRH deficiency (when associated with anosmia: Kallmann's syndrome), other genetic mutations, e.g. DAX1 (associated with congenital adrenal hypoplasia), HESX1 (associated with septo-optic dysplasia), isolated LH or FSH deficiency
Other causes of hypopituitarism: vascular/infection, etc. (*See* Hypopituitarism)

Hyperprolactinaemia

Systemic diseases

Cystic fibrosis
Crohn's disease/ulcerative colitis, malnutrition of any cause
Cirrhosis
Chronic renal failure
Thalassaemia: → repeated blood transfusions → haemosiderosis and hypothalamic dysfunction

Rare causes

Laurence–Moon–Beidl syndrome
Prader–Willi syndrome

Male
1° hypogonadism (hypergonadotrophic):
Gonadal dysgensis
Klinefelter's syndrome (XXY): testes are small and firm with dysgenetic
seminiferous tubules
Cryptorchism: undescended testes
Anorchia: Vanishing testis syndrome: testicular tissue present in fetal life but
absent in the adult

Gonadal damage
Infection (e.g. mumps, echovirus, group B arbovirus, lymphocytic
choriomeningitis),
Trauma, torsion
Autoimmune
Surgery (orchidectomy)
Radiation
Drugs/toxins: cyclophosphamide
Alcohol, marijuana, heroin: ↓ testosterone levels
Genetic mutations
LH/FSH b subunits, LH receptor, FSH receptor, defects in enzymes involved in
testosterone synthesis, myotonic dystrophy

2° hypogonadism (hypogonadotrophic):
Hypopituitarism
Pituitary tumour/surgery/radiation/infiltrations; See Hypopituitarism
Congenital GnRH deficiency (idiopathic hypogonadotrophic hypogonadism)
(Kallmann's syndrome: GnRH deficiency + one or more non-gonadal
congenital abnormalities e.g. anosmia), other genetic mutations, e.g. DAX1,
HESX1, Prop-1

Hyperprolactinaemia
Systemic diseases
Cystic fibrosis
Crohn's disease/ulcerative colitis, malnutrition of any cause
Cirrhosis
Chronic renal failure
Thalassaemia: → repeated blood transfusions → haemosiderosis and
hypothalamic dysfunction

Rare causes
Laurence–Moon–Beidl syndrome
Prader–Willi syndrome

Hypokalaemia
Gastrointestinal loss
Vomiting, diarrhoea, villous adenoma, VIPoma, fistulae, ileostomies

Renal loss
Excess mineralocortcoids (→↑ K^+ excretion)
Hyperaldosteronism
↑↑ Glucocorticoids: Cushing's syndrome, liquorice (inhibits 11 β-hydroxysteroid
dehydrogenase and ↓ glucocorticoid metabolism), 11 β-hydroxysteroid
dehydrogenase deficiency
Congenital adrenal hyperplasia (11 β-hydroxylase and 17 α-hydroxylase
deficiency)

Hypokalaemia continued
↑ Na⁺ delivery to distal nephron (→↑ Na⁺ absorption and K⁺ secretion)
Osmotic diuresis (e.g. in glycosuria)
Diuretics: thiazides and loop diuretics (also ↑ aldosterone secretion)
Bartter's syndrome, Gitelman's syndrome

Others
Hypomagnesaemia
Renal tubular acidosis (type I & II)
Renal tubular damage
Liddle's syndrome (autosomal dominant condition, primary ↑ in collecting tubule
    sodium reabsorption and often potassium secretion)

Redistribution into the cells
Insulin, β-agonists, alkalosis

Hypomagnesaemia
↓ **Intake or GI losses:** malnutrition, alcoholism, diarrhoea, malabsorption,
    intestinal resection, intestinal fistulae
Renal losses:
    Diuretics (loop and thiazides)
    Alcohol abuse
    Drugs: nephrotoxins, e.g. aminoglycosides, amphotericin B, cyclosporine,
        cisplatin
    Diabetes mellitus, hypercalcaemia, hyperthyroidism, hyperaldosteronism,
        tubular dysfunction (post-acute tubular necrosis, postobstructive diuresis,
        Bartter's or Gitelman's syndrome)
Other: Post-operative, post-parathyroidectomy, pancreatitis (acute), foscarnet

Hyponatraemia
Pseudohyponatraemia:
    Hyperproteinaemia (e.g. multiple myeloma), hypertriglyceridaemia
    Hyperglycaemia
Artifactual: taking blood from the arm into which low sodium solution is infused
Hypervolaemic (oedematous) patients:
    Cirrohsis, CCF, nephrotic syndrome, renal failure (urine Na⁺>20)
Hypovolaemic (dehydrated) patients:
    Renal loss (urine Na⁺>20): Diuretics (thiazides), renal tubular acidosis, salt-
        losing nephropathy, adrenal insufficiency
    Extra-renal loss (urine Na⁺<20): diarrhoea, vomiting, burns, pancreatitis
Euvolaemic patients:
    Hypothyroidism, adrenal insufficiency, SIADH

Hypoparathyroidism
See Hypocalcaemia

Hypophosphataemia
Redistribution into cells
↑ Insulin, e.g. recovery from diabetic ketoacidosis (treatment with insulin
    stimulates glycolysis and phosphate uptake by the cells), refeeding (e.g. in
    alcoholics)
Respiratory alkalosis (alkalosis stimulates glycolysis and phosphate uptake by the
    cells)
Hungry bone syndrome (following parathyroidectomy in patients with pre-
    existing osteopenia): due to marked deposition of Ca^{2+} and phosphate in bone

Gastrointestinal

Phosphate binders, e.g. aluminum/magnesium-containing antacids
Diarrhoea (chronic)
↓ Dietary intake

Renal

Hyperparathyroidism (1° & 2°):↑ urinary excretion
Vitamin D deficiency/resistance (both by ↓ GI absorption and by causing
  hypocalcaemia and 2° hyperparathyroidism)
Hereditary hypophosphataemic rickets (X-linked, autosomal dominant), tumour-
  induced osteomalacia
Osmotic diuresis, e.g. glycosuria
Fanconi syndrome

Hypopyon

Infection: endophthalmitis, corneal ulcers
Inflammation: anterior uveitis (See Uveitis)
Malignancy: necrosis of intraocular tumours/metastases (e.g. leukaemia,
  lymphoma, retinoblastoma)
Trauma, surgery

Hypopigmented macules

Post-inflammatory
Vitiligo
Tinea versicolor
Halo naevus
Sarcoidosis
Tuberous sclerosis
T-cell lymphoma (cutaneous)
Leprosy

Hypopituitarism

Pituitary tumour
Pituitary surgery/radiation
Infection: meningitis/encephalitis, syphilis (rare)
Inflammation/infiltration: TB, sarcoidosis, lymphoma, abscess, histiocytosis X,
  haemochromatosis, lymphocytic hypophysitis
Vascular: pituitary apoplexy (infarction/haemorrhage), Sheehan's syndrome
Hypothalamic: anorexia, severe exercise, starvation
Mutations: e.g. Pit-1, Prop-1

Hyposplenism

See Howell–Jolly bodies

Hypotension

Septicaemia
Hypovolaemia:
  Haemorrhage
  GI loss
  Renal loss (diuretic, diabetes mellitus, diabetes insipidus, post-obstructive
    diuresis, acute renal failure
  Cutaneous loss (exudative lesions, burns)
Adrenal insufficiency
Cardiovascular:
  Any condition that ↓ cardiac output, e.g. arrhythmias, ↓ diastolic filling
    (pericardial disease), myocardial disease, outflow obstruction

Hypotension continued
Postural hypotension
Volume depletion
Autonomic neuropathy:
  Metabolic: diabetes mellitus, amyloidosis (rare), drugs (tricyclics, L-dopa)
  Inflammation: Guillain–Barré syndrome
  Infection: HIV, syphilis
  Tumours: paraneoplastic (e.g. small cell lung cancer), hypothalamic
  Degenerative: Parkinson's disease, multiple system atrophy, Shy–Drager
    syndrome
  Familial dysautonomia (Riley–Day syndrome)
Drugs: Antihypertensives, diuretics, nitrates, antidepressants, sedatives
Leg vein insufficiency

Hypothyroidism
Primary
Congenital: athyreosis, dyshormogenesis, iodide deficiency
Acquired:
  Autoimmune (Hashimoto's thyroiditis)
  Iatrogenic (surgery, radio-iodine, drugs, e.g. amiodarone, Lithium,
    thionamides)
  Iodide deficiency/excess

Secondary
Hypothalamic/pituitary disease

I

Impotence
Psychological (patients may have morning erections)
Drugs: alcohol, antidepressants, β-blockers, cannabis, diuretics (spirinolactone), major tranquilizers
Endocrine disorders: hypogonadism/androgen deficiency, hyperthyroidism, prolactinomas, acromegaly
Neurological: autonomic neuropathy (e.g. diabetes mellitus, uraemia), nerve damage after bladder neck/prostate surgery, multiple sclerosis
Vascular disease (e.g. atherosclerosis)

Incontinence
Urinary: See Urinary incontinence
Faecal: See Faecal incontinence

Indigestion
See Dyspepsia

Infertility
Female
Anovulation (1°/2° hypogonadism)
Obstructed fallopian tubes (e.g. post- infection/inflammation/surgery: adhesions)
Uterine cavity abnormalities (e.g. fibroids, endometriosis)
Chromosome abnormalities
Antiphospholipid syndrome
(Note: semen analysis (sperm density, motility etc.) should be performed to exclude male factor infertility.)

Male
Hypogonadism (1° or 2°)
Varicocoele
Immotile sperms
Obstruction of epididymis, vas deferens
Coital disorders

Insomnia
Self-limiting: stress, travel etc.
Psychological: depression, mania, anxiety
Medical: drugs, withdrawal of antidepressants/hypnotics, caffeine, pain, pruritus, nocturia, asthma, alcoholism, apnoea, tinnitus, dystonia

Internuclear ophthalmoplegia
Involvement of medial longitudinal fasciculus in the brainstem:
Multiple sclerosis
Vascular: infarction, haemorrhage
Gliomas
Wernicke's encephalopathy

Intracranial pressure, ↑
Vascular: haemorrhage (extradural, subdural, subarachnoid, intracerebral)
Infection: meningitis/encephalitis, abscess
Trauma: head injury

Intracranial pressure, ↑ continued
Tumours
Benign intracranial hypertension, hydrocephalus, cerebral oedema

Iritis
See Uveitis

Iron deficiency
See Anaemia, microcytic

Iron overload
Repeated transfusions, e.g. thalassaemia
Haemochromatosis
Iron therapy

J

Jaccoud's arthropathy
SLE
Rheumatic fever
Bronchial carcinoma
Hypocomplementaemic urticarial vasculitis

Jaundice
Pre-hepatic
Haemolysis (*See* Anaemia, haemolytic), ineffective erythropoiesis,
  ↓ glucuronidation (Gilbert's syndrome, Crigler–Najjar syndrome)

Hepatocellular
Viral: A, B, C; (other infections: CMV, EBV, toxoplasmosis, leptospirosis, Q fever)
Drugs (paracetamol, anti-TB drugs, statins, sodium valproate, halothane), toxins,
  herbal medications
Alcoholic hepatitis
Autoimmune hepatitis
Cirrhosis, hepatic metastases, hepatic abscess
Wilson's disease, haemochromatosis, α1-antitrypsin deficiency, Budd–Chiari
  syndrome
Septicaemia
Dubin–Johnson syndrome, Rotor syndrome

Obstructive
Gallstones (in the common bile duct)
Carcinoma of head of pancreas/ampulla of Vater/bile duct
Lymphadenopathy at the porta hepatic
Benign stricture (following invasive procedures)
Drugs: (antibiotics, OCPs, chlorpromazine, sulphonylureas, gold)
Primary sclerosing cholangitis, primary biliary cirrhosis
Parasites, e.g. schistosomiasis/fasciola, pancreatitis, AIDS cholangiopathy

Jugular foramen syndrome (involving cranial nerves IX, X and XI)
Meningiomata
Metastases
Neurofibroma of IXth, Xth or XIIth nerves
Other tumours: cerebellopontine angle tumours, cholesteatomas, glomus
  tumour, carotid body tumour
Trauma: fracture at base of skull
Infection from the middle ear spreading into the posterior fossa
Jugular vein thrombosis
Paget's disease

Jugular venous pressure
↑ JVP
Right heart failure
Tricuspid regurgitation
Pericardial effusion, constrictive pericarditis
Fluid overload
Obstruction of superior vena cava

Jugular venous pressure continued
'a' waves (Cannon waves)

Regular: nodal rhythm, paroxysmal nodal tachycardia, partial heart block with very long PR interval

Irregular: complete heart block, multiple ectopic beats

K

KCCT
See APTT, ↑

Ketonuria
Diabetes
Starvation
↑ Metabolic requirements: fever, pregnancy, thyrotoxicosis
Glycogen storage diseases

Kidney, enlarged
Cystic kidney
Carcinoma
Hydronephrosis, pyonephrosis
Hypertrophy (following contralateral nephretomy)
Perirenal haematoma
Congenital anomaly

Knee, painful/swollen
See Monoarthralgia

Knee, swelling
Septic arthritis (staphylococci, gonococci, Gram −ve bacilli, TB, Lyme disease)
Trauma, haemarthrosis (in haemophiliacs)
Gout/pseudogout
Rheumatoid arthritis, osteoarthritis
Seronegative arthritides (reactive arthritis, enteropathic arthritis (IBD, Whipple's
    disease), ankylosing spondylitis, psoriatic arthritis)
Systemic: SLE, Sjögren's syndrome, sarcoidosis, Behçet's disease, vasculitides
Malignancy
Localized swellings:
    Anterior: pre-patellar bursa
    Infrapatellar bursa
    Osgood–Schlatter disease
    Lateral/medial: lateral/medial meniscus cyst
    Exostosis
    Posterior:
    Semimembranous bursa
    Baker's cyst
    Popliteal aneurysm

Koebner phenomenon
Psoriasis
Lichen planus
Molluscum contagiosum
Warts
Vitiligo

Kussmaul's breathing
Metabolic acidosis, e.g. diabetic ketoacidosis, uraemia, etc.

Kussmaul's sign

Pericardial effusion
Constrictive pericarditis
Restrictive cardiomyopathy

L

Lactate dehydrogenase
Myocardial infarction
Haemolysis
Hepatocyte damage
Pulmonary embolism
Tumour necrosis

Leg pain
Vascular: arterial occlusion: acute (thromboembolism, trauma, e.g. fracture),
　chronic (arterosclerosis, arteritis, Buerger's disease)
　　DVT
Neurological: lumbar canal stenosis
　Radiculopathy, plexopathy
　Peripheral neuropathy
Musculoskeletal: soft-tissue (muscle, tendon, ligament) injury, muscle spasm
Arthritis

Leg swelling
Bilateral
Heart failure
Liver failure, other causes of hypoalbuminaemia (malnutrition, malabsorption,
　nephrotic syndrome, protein-losing enteropathy)
Renal failure
Hypothyroidism
Iatrogenic: oestrogens, calcium channel blockers, fluid overload
Venous insufficiency: acute (prolonged sitting), chronic
Venous obstruction, e.g. pelvic mass, pregnancy, IVC/bilateral iliac vein
　obstruction

Unilateral
Acute
DVT
Cellulitis
Compartment syndrome, trauma
Baker's cyst rupture

Chronic
Varicose veins
Lymphoedema (non-pitting): primary, lymph node involvement: radiotherapy,
　infection (filariasis), malignant infiltration, excision
Immobility

Leg weakness
See Weak legs

Leukaemoid reaction
Severe infection, TB
Burns
Malignant bone marrow infiltration
Haemolysis
Haemorrhage

Leukoerythroblastic anaemia
Marrow infiltration, e.g. malignancy
Hypoxia
Severe anaemia

Leukoplakia
Trauma/friction
Infection: HIV, candida, syphilis

Livedo reticularis
Cryoglobulinaemia, systemic lupus erythematosus, antiphospholipid syndrome,
    polyarteritis nodosa
Cholesterol embolus

Lip swellings
Insect bite
Allergic/anaphylactic reaction
Angioneurotic shock (C1 esterase deficiency)
Crohn's disease
Sarcoid
Granulomatous cheilitis

Lip erosions
Herpes simplex
Pemphigus
Erythema multiforme/Stephens–Johnson syndrome
Impetigo

Lipodystrophy, partial
Partial
Congenital
HIV drugs: protease inhibitors
Associated with membranoproliferative glomerulonephritis (type II)

Local
Idiopathic
Injection, e.g. insulin
Pressure
Panniculitis

Liver function tests
AST (SGOT), ↑
Hepatocyte damage (See Jaundice)
Haemolysis
Myocardial infarction
Skeletal muscle damage

ALT (SGPT), ↑
Hepatocyte damage
Shock

ALP, ↑
Liver disease: cholestasis (See Jaundice, obstructive)

Bone disease ($\uparrow$ osteoblastic activity): growth in adolescence, healing fracture, Paget's disease of bone, osteomalacia, bone metastases, hyperparathyroidism, renal failure
Placenta: pregnancy
Small intestinal disease

Loss of consciousness
See Blackouts

Lower motor neurone lesions
Examples include:
    Anterior horn cell: motor neurone disease, poliomyelitis
    Spinal root: cervical and lumbar disc protrusion
    Peripheral nerves: trauma, entrapment, mononeuritis multiplex, polyneuropathy
See also Cranial nerve palsies

Lung function tests
Obstructive defect: FEV$_1$/FVC ratio $< 75\%$
Asthma
COPD

Restrictive defect: FEV$_1$/FVC ratio $> 75\%$
Pulmonary fibrosis:
    Cryptogenic fibrosing alveolitis
    Connective tissue diseases: scleroderma, SLE, sarcoidosis, rheumatoid arthritis, ankylosing spondylitis
    Drugs (amiodarone, busulphan, bleomycin, nitrofurantoin), radiation
    Extrinsic allergic alveolitis (e.g. Farmers' lung, Bird fancier's lung, Malt worker's lung)
    Pneumoconioses (Coal workers' pneumoconiosis, asbestosis, silicosis, berylliosis)

Transfer factor
$\downarrow$
Interstitial lung disease (pulmonary fibrosis)
Pulmonary embolus
Emphysema
Anaemia
Arteriovenous malformation

$\uparrow$
Pulmonary haemorrhage
Polycythaemia
Pneumonectomy
Asthma
L $\rightarrow$ R shunt
Severe obesity, exercise prior to the test session

Lymphadenopathy
Infection:
    Bacterial, TB, less commonly: brucellosis, syphilis, cat scratch disease
    Viral (e.g. HIV, EBV, CMV, rubella, measles)
    Toxoplasmosis, filariasis, fungal (e.g. coccidiomycosis)

Lymphadenopathy continued

Inflammatory/connective tissue disease: rheumatoid arthritis, sarcoidosis, SLE
Malignancy: metastases, lymphoma, leukaemia
Rare: thyrotoxicosis, histiocytosis, psoriasis, eczema, phenytoin

Lymphocytosis

See White cell count

Lymphopenia

See White cell count

M

Macroglossia

Hypothyroidism
Amyloidosis
Acromegaly
Mucopolysaccharidosis
Down's syndrome
Chronic infections, e.g. TB
Space-occupying lesions, e.g. rhabdomyosarcomas

Masses and swellings

Abdomen

Right hypochondrium

Hepatomegaly (*See* Hepatomegaly)
Enlarged gallbladder (empyema, mucocele, obstruction of the common bile duct
   e.g. pancreatic cancer, gallbladder mass)
Enlarged kindey (*See* Kidney, enlarged)
Colonic mass

Epigastrium

Gastric carcinoma
Pancreatic mass: carcinoma, pseudocyst
Liver: left lobe, post-necrotic nodule of a cirrhotic liver
Large recti

Left hypochondrium

Splenomegaly
Enlarged kidney
Pancreatic cancer

Right iliac fossa

Carcinoma of caecum
Crohn's disease
Appendix mass
TB (ileocaecal)
Iliac lymphadenopathy
Ovarian cyst
Transplanted pelvic kidney

Left iliac fossa

Loaded sigmoid colon (esp. in constipation)
Diverticular disease
Colonic cancer
Crohn's disease
Iliac lymphadenopathy
Ovarian cyst
Transplanted pelvic kidney

Suprapubic

Enlarged bladder
Pregnant uterus
Fibroids
Ovarian cyst

Masses and swellings continued

Inguinal
Hernias (inguinal, femoral)
Lymphadenopathy
Vascular: saphena varix, femoral aneurysm
Psoas abscess
Ectopic/undescended testis
Lipoma of the cord
Hydrocoele of the cord

Scrotal
Indirect inguinal hernia
Hydrocele
Epididymal cyst
Spermatocoele
Testicular tumour
Gumma
Painful swellings (See Testicular pain and swelling)

Megacolon
Inflammatory bowel disease
Ischaemic colitis
Pseudomembranous colitis
Amoebic colitis
CMV colitis (in patients with HIV infection/AIDS)
Trypanosomiasis (South American)

Memory loss
See Amnesia

Menorrhagia
Local anatomical disorders: fibroids, polyps (uterine and cervical), adenomyosis, endometriosis, malignancy (cervical, endometrial, ovarian), chronic pelvic infection
Systemic problems: hyperthyroidism, coagulopathies (e.g. von Willebrand's disease), anticoagulants
Dysfunctional uterine bleeding

Menstrual bleeding, irregular
Similar causes as Menorrhagia

Methaemoglobinaemia
Drugs: dapsone, nitrates, nitrites, primaquine, quinolones, sulfasalazine
Congenital

Miosis
Reactive to light
Old age
Horner's syndrome

Non–reactive
Drugs: pilocarpine eye drops, opiates
Argyll Robertson pupil (irregular pupils)
Anterior uveitis ($\uparrow$ pupil light reflex)
Pontine lesion

Mitral regurgitation
Rheumatic heart disease
Infective endocarditis
Mitral valve prolapse
Papillary muscle rupture (after MI) or dysfunction (ischaemic heart disease/
    cardiomyopathy)
Chordal rupture and floppy mitral valve associated with connective tissue
    diseases (pseudoxanthoma elasticum, osteogenesis imperfecta, Ehlers–Danlos
    syndrome, Marfan's syndrome, SLE)
Functional mitral regurgitation: secondary to left ventricular dilatation

Mitral stenosis
Rheumatic heart disease (90%)
Less common: congenital, calcified mitral valve ring, carcinoid, endocarditis,
    mucopolysaccharidoses, prosthetic valve

Monoarthralgia
Articular
Infection: septic arthritis (staphylococci, gonococci, Gram –ve bacilli, TB, Lyme
    disease)
Trauma, haemarthrosis (haemophilia)
Gout/pseudogout
Rheumatoid arthritis, osteoarthritis
Seronegative arthritides (reactive arthritis, enteropathic arthritis (IBD, Whipple's
    disease), ankylosing spondylitis, psoriatic arthritis)
Systemic: SLE, Sjögren's syndrome, sarcoidosis, Behçet's disease, vasculitides
Malignancy

Extra-articular
Bursitis, tenosynovitis, cellulitis

Monocytosis
See White Cell Count

Mononeuritis multiplex
Infection: HIV, herpes zoster, Lyme disease, leprosy
Inflammation: vasculitis (primary, e.g. PAN, Wegener's granulomatosis, Churg–
    Strauss syndrome, cryoglobulinaemia; secondary: rheumatoid arthritis, SLE),
    sarcoidosis, Sjögren's syndrome, Behçet's disease
Metabolic: diabetes mellitus
Malignancy: infiltration (lymphoma, carcinoma)
Hereditary neuropathy: prone to pressure palsies?

Mouth ulcers
See Ulcers

Murmurs
Systolic
Ejection systolic:
    Aortic area: aortic stenosis (See Aortic stenosis), aortic sclerosis
    Pulmonary area: innocent, atrial septal defect, pulmonary stenosis
    (Note: in HOCM an ejection systolic murmur is heard at left sternal border,
    radiating to aortic and mitral areas)

Murmurs continued

Pansystolic:
Mitral regurgitation (*See* Mitral regurgitation), ventricular septal defect, tricuspid regurgitation (*See* Tricuspid regurgitation)

Diastolic

Early diastolic: aortic regurgitation (*See* Aortic regurgitation), pulmonary regurgitation
Mid-systolic: mitral stenosis (*See* Mitral stenosis), tricuspid stenosis (rare)
Continuous: patent ductus arteriosus

Myalgia

Myopathy: metabolic, inflammatory, infective, drugs, alcohol (*See* Proximal muscle weakness)
Muscle haematoma, abscess
Infection: systemic
Inflammatory/connective tissue disease
Malignancy
Malignant hyperpyrexia
Parkinson's disease
Polymyalgia rheumatica
Fibromyalgia
Chronic fatigue syndrome

Mydriasis

Drugs: mydriatic eye drops (antimuscarinics, e.g. atropine, cyclopentolate, tropicamide), overdose (cocaine, amphetamine, glutethamide), poisoning, e.g. belladonna
Trauma: post-traumatic iridoplegia, iridectomy, lens implant
Third nerve palsy
Holmes–Adie pupil (degeneration of the nerve to the ciliary ganglion)
Acute angle closure glaucoma
Deep coma, cerebral death

Myoclonus

Congenital
Acute metabolic encephalopathy
Creutzfeldt–Jakob disease
Alzheimer's disease
Lysosomal storage diseases, e.g. Gaucher's disease, Tay–Sachs disease

Myoglobinuria

Trauma, surgery
Ischaemia, immobility, coma
Rigorous exercise, seizures
Myositis
Metabolic: hypokalaemia, hypophosphataemia
Drugs/toxins: fibrates, statins, alcohol, CO
Others: malignant hyperthermia, neuroleptic malignant syndrome, inherited muscle disorders

N

Nail pitting
Psoriasis
Alopecia areata
Eczema
Lichen Planus
Trauma

Eczema
Lichen planus
Trauma
Nasal discharge
Allergic rhinitis: seasonal/perennial
Vasomotor rhinitis
Infection: viral (acute/chronic), sinusitis
   Rarely: TB, fungal, syphilis, AIDS
Inflammation: polyps (e.g. cystic fibrosis), Wegener's granulomatosis, sarcoidosis,
   midline granuloma
Trauma: foreign body, fracture of anterior fossa (CSF leak)
Tumours (nasopharyngeal, maxillary sinus)

Nausea
See Vomiting

Neck pain
Postural, cold exposure
Trauma: acute flexion-extension injury, fracture, dislocation
Degenerative: cervical spondylosis, diffuse idiopathic skeletal hyperostosis
Inflammatory: rheumatoid arthritis, spondylarthropathy, polymyalgia
   rheumatica
Neurological: disc prolapse, meningism (meningitis, subarachnoid haemorrhage),
   vertebral/carotid artery dissection, brachial plexus lesions (trauma, thoracic
   outlet syndrome)
Infection: osteomyelitis (e.g. TB), discitis, general systemic infection (cervical
   myalgia)
Malignancy: primary and secondary bone tumours, myeloma
Metabolic/endocrine: osteoporosis, osteomalacia, Paget's disease of bone,
   thyroiditis, haemorrhagic thyroid cyst
Referred pain: temporomandibular/acromioclavicular joint, shoulder, pharynx,
   heart/vessels, lung, diaphragm

Neck swellings
Midline
Thyroid gland swelling
Thyroglossal cyst
Lymph nodes
Rare: sublingual dermoid cyst, pharyngeal pouch, plunging ranula, subhyoid
   bursa, laryngeal/tracheal/oesophageal carcinoma
Manubrium swelling:
   Soft: lipoma
   Hard: bony tumour or plasmacytoma
   Pulsatile: eroding aortic aneurysm

Neck swellings continued
Anterior triangle
Lymph nodes, cold abscess (TB)
Salivary gland (submandibular/parotid) swelling
Branchial cyst
Carotid body tumour
Carotid body aneurysm
Sternomastoid tumour

Posterior triangle
Lymph nodes, cold abscess (TB)
Cystic hygroma
Subclavian artery aneurysm
Tumour of clavicle

Nerve thickening (hypertrophy)
Tuberculoid leprosy
Sarcoidosis
Amyloidosis
Neurofibromatosis
Acromegaly
Hereditary sensorimotor neuropathy type 1
Refsum's disease

Neutropenia
See White cell count

Neutrophilia
See White cell count

Night sweats
Infections: chronic infections, e.g. TB, subacute bacterial infections (e.g.
    endocarditis, osteomyelitis), others: HIV, histoplasmosis
Malignancy, e.g. lymphoma, solid tumours
Menopause
Medications: GnRH agonists, antidepressants

Nipple discharge
Milky: late pregnancy, lactation, puberty, hyperprolactinaemia
purulent: mastitis, breast abscess, TB (rare)
Yellow/green: duct ectasia, fibrocystic disease
Blood-stained: intraductal carcinoma, intraductal papilloma, Paget's disease of
    the nipple

Nocturia
See Frequency

Normoblasts
Marrow infiltration
Haemolysis
Hypoxia

Nystagmus
Physiological: at the extreme lateral gaze
Pendular (to-and-fro movements have equal velocity): congenital

Jerky (slow-phase and fast phase are present):
  Acute labyrinthitis, other inner ear (labyrinth/vestibular nerve) diseases, e.g.
  Ménière's disease, benign positional vertigo (otoconial debris in semicircular
  canals), vestibular neuronitis, acoustic neuroma
  Brainstem/vestibular nuclei: vascular (CVA), inflammation (multiple sclerosis,
  tumour), toxic (alcoholism)
  Cerebellar disease (*See* Cerebellar signs)
  Drugs (e.g. phenytoin)
Nystagmus is also seen in internuclear ophthalmoplegia (↓ adduction on the side
  of lesion, nystagmus of the contralateral abducting eye)

Note: In **A**: hearing loss, tinnitus and vertigo may be present, past phase is to the
  contralateral side of the lesion. In **C** other cerebellar signs are present, fast
  phase is to the side of the lesion.

Rotatory nystagmus: a lesion in labyrinth or brainstem
Vertical nystagmus: drugs or brainstem lesion. If down-beating on downgaze:
  localizes to the region of the foramen magnum

O

Ocular pain
Pain on eye movement
Optic neuritis
Orbital myositis
See Painful red eye

Oedema, ankle
Pitting, bilateral
Heart failure
Liver failure, other causes of hypoalbuminaemia: malnutrition, malabsorption,
    nephrotic syndrome, protein-losing enteropathy
Renal failure
Hypothyroidism
Iatrogenic: oestrogens, calcium channel blockers, fluid overload
Venous insufficiency: acute (prolonged sitting), chronic
Venous obstruction, e.g. pelvic mass, pregnancy, IVC/bilateral iliac vein
    obstruction

Non-pitting
Lymphoedema: primary, lymph node involvement: **r**adiotherapy, **i**nfection
    (filariasis), **m**alignant infiltration, **e**xcision

Oliguria
Dehydration
Renal failure (acute, chronic): pre-renal (e.g. shock), renal (acute tubular
    necrosis), post-renal (stones, tumour, retroperitoneal fibrosis)

Onycholysis
Psoriasis
Fungal infection
Thyrotoxicosis
Trauma
Tetracyclines

Optic disc
Atrophy
Optic neuritis (MS)
↑ Intracranial **p**ressure: 2° to long-standing papilloedema (e.g. tumours)
Toxic/metabolic/drugs: tobacco, alcohol, vitamin B_{12} deficiency, diabetes,
    ethambutol
Infection/infiltration: spread from sinuses, syphilis, sarcoid
Compression: intra-orbital (e.g. optic nerve tumours), tumour of pituitary or
    sphenoid sinus, carotid aneurysm
Anterior ischaemic optic neuropathy
Trauma: orbital fracture, indirect trauma
Retinal disease: retinitis pigmentosa, macular degeneration
Occlusion of retinal artery
↑ **P**ressure inside the eye (glaucoma)
Hereditary: Leber's optic atrophy, hereditary ataxias, e.g. Friedreich's, DIDMOAD*

*Diabetes insipidus, diabetes mellitus, optic atrophy, deafness.

Blurred
Paplloedema:

↑ Intracranial pressure: Haemorrhage (extradural, subdural, subarachnoid, intracerebral), head injury. Meningitis/encephalitis, tumours, abscesses, benign intracranial hypertension, hydrocephalus, cerebral oedema
Malignant hypertension
Retinal vein thrombosis, venous sinus thrombosis
Hypercapnia
Hypoparathyroidism
Hypervitaminosis A
Lead poisoning

Papillitis (demyelination)

Oral pigmentation
Racial (African, Asian)
Post-trauma/inflammation
Peutz–Jegher's syndrome
Addison's disease
Acanthosis nigricans
Fixed drug eruptions
Heavy metal poisoning

Oral ulcers
See Ulcers

Osler nodes
Subacute bacterial endocarditis
SLE
Haemolytic anaemia
Gonococcal infection

Otorrhoea
Watery: eczema of the ear canal, CSF
Mucoid: chronic suppuirative otitis media with a perforation
Purulent: acute otitis externa
Mucopurulent/bloody: trauma, carcinoma of the ear, acute otitis media
Foul smelling: chronic suppurative otitis media with cholasteatoma

Oxygen saturation, sources of errors
Hypoperfusion (e.g. shock)
Improper probe placement
Intensive ambient light
Motion artifact
MRI
Nail polish
Skin pigmentation
Abnormal haemoglobins: carboxyhaemoglobin, methaemoglobin
Venous congestion/pulsations: e.g. tricuspid valve incompetence

P

P wave
Absent
Atrial fibrillation
Hyperkalaemia
Sinoatrial block, junctional (AV nodal) rhythm

Tall
Pulmonary hypertension (primary, secondary to pulmonary emboli, COPD)
Pulmonary stenosis
Tricuspid stenosis

Painful red eye
Scleritis
Anterior uveitis
Acute angle closure glaucoma
Corneal ulcer/bacterial keratitis

Pallor
Racial, familial
Shock
Syncope
Anaemia
Endocrine: hypothyroidism, hypopituitarism
Other: albinism, vitiligo (widespread), phenylketonuria

Palmar erythema
Liver disease
Alcoholism
Rheumatoid arthritis
Thyrotoxicosis
Pregnancy
Chronic leukaemia

Palmoplantar hyperkeratosis
See Hyperkeratosis

Palmoplantar rash
Palmar erythema (*see above*)
Pompholyx eczema
Palmoplantar pustulosis (may be associated with synovitis, acne, hyperostosis and
    osteitis in SAPHO syndrome)
Reiter's syndrome (keratoderma blenorrhagica)
Janeway lesions (infective endocarditis)
Secondary syphilis
Erythema multiforme
Sign of graft-versus-host disease

Palpitations
Fever, exercise, anaemia, pregnancy
Drugs (caffeine, nicotine, salbutamol, anticholinergics, vasodilators, cocaine)
Cardiac: any arrhythmia* (e.g. AF, extrasystoles, SVT, VT), pacemaker, valvular
    disease, cardiac shunts, cardiomyopathy, atrial myxoma

Endocrine: hyperthyroidism, phaeochromocytomas, hypoglycaemia,
    mastocytosis
Psychiatric: panic attacks, generalized anxiety disorder, depression,
    somatization

* See Tachycardia.

Pancytopenia
Aplastic anaemia
    Congenital: Fanconi's
    Radiation
    Chemicals: benzene, insecticides
    Drugs: chloramphenicol, cytotoxics, gold
    Infection: HIV, viral hepatitis, measles
    Idiopathic
Megaloblastic anaemia
Marrow infiltration
    Lymphoma
    Leukaemia (acute)
    Metastasis
    Myeloma
    Myelofibrosis
SLE, sepsis, hypersplenism, paroxysmal nocturnal haemoglobinuria (PNH)

Papilloedema
See Optic disc

Pappenheimer bodies
Sideroblastic anaemia
Haemolytic anaemia
Post-splenectomy

Paraesthesiae
Peripheral neuropathy, e.g. diabetes mellitus, alcoholism etc. (See
    Polyneuropathy)
Peripheral nerve entrapment/compression, e.g. cervical rib, carpal tunnel
    syndrome, disc herniation
Spinal cord disease, e.g. cord/nerve root compression, multiple sclerosis
Rarely: cortical/thalamic lesions
Hypocalcaemia, e.g. in respiratory alkalosis, hypomagnesaemia

Paraproteinaemia
Multiple myeloma
Waldenström's macroglobulinaemia
Primary amyloidosis
Monoclonal gammopathy (benign paraproteinaemia)
Lymphoma, leukaemia
Heavy chain disease

Parotid enlargement
Bilateral
Sjögren's syndrome
Sarcoidosis
Lymphoma
Anorexia

Parotid enlargement continued
Acromegaly
Alcoholics
Diabetics, hypertriglyceridaemia
Infection: mumps, HIV

Unilateral
Tumours, e.g. benign mixed parotid tumour, Warthin's tumour
Calculi
Cysts
Bacterial infection

Pathological fractures
Congenital: osteogenesis imperfecta, fibrous dysplasia
Malignancy: primary, secondary, myeloma
Osteomyelitis
Osteoporosis
Osteomalacia
Paget's disease of bone
Benign tumours: bone cysts, chondroma

Pelvic girdle pain
Degenerative disc disease (with facet impingement or nuclear prolapse)
Osteoarthritis of hip
Sacroiliitis
Trochanteric bursitis
Meralgia paraesthesia

Percussion note
Dull
Pleural effusion (stony dull)
Collapse
Consolidation
Fibrosis
Pleural thickening

Hyper-resonant
Pneumothorax
COPD (hyperinflation)

Pericarditis
Idiopathic
Infection (viral, e.g. coxsackie, EBV, varicella, mumps, HIV; bacterial, e.g.
    Streptococcus, TB; fungal)
Inflammatory/connective tissue diseases: rheumatoid arthritis, SLE
Myocardial infarction
Malignancy
Myxoedema
Uraemia
Radiotherapy
Surgery/trauma
Drugs: hydralazine, isoniazid

Pericardial effusion
See Pericarditis

Pericardial rub
See Pericarditis

Periorbital oedema
See Facial swelling

Peripheral oedema
See Oedema

Pes cavus
Charcot–Marie–Tooth disease
Friedreich's ataxia
Poliomyelitis
Spina bifida
Syringomyelia
Homocysteinuria

Petechiae
See Purpura

Photodistributed rash
Drugs, e.g. amiodarone, sulphonamides, tetracyclines, griseofulvin,
    phenothiazines, chloroquine
SLE
Dermatomyositis
Porphyria cutanea tarda
Pellagra
Polymorphous light eruption

Pigmentation
See Hyperpigmentation and Hypopigmented macules

Pins and needles
See Paraesthesiae

Platelets
↓ **Production**
Bone marrow failure
Myeloma, myelofibrosis, marrow infiltration (lymphoma, carcinoma), anaemia
    (megaloblastic, aplastic), leukaemia
Drugs: (cytotoxics, chloramphenicol, alcohol), radiotherapy
↓ Megakaryocytes: chemicals, drugs (e.g. co-trimoxazole), viral infection

↑ **Destruction/consumption**
Autoimmune (ITP)
SLE, CLL, lymphoma
Infections (malaria, viral, e.g. HIV)
Drugs (e.g. analgesics, antibiotics, anticonvulsant, anti-diabetics, heparin,
    quinine, quinidine)
DIC, TTP, HUS
Sequestration: splenic pooling due to splenomegaly
Dilutional loss (massive transfusion of stored blood)
Artifactual: blood clotting in the sample

Platelets continued
Functional disorders
Bernard–Soulier disease
Glanzmann's thrombasthenia
Storage pool disease
Liver disease, myeloproliferative disorders, paraproteinaemia, aspirin, uraemia

↑ Platelets (thrombocytosis)
Secondary
Blood loss
Infection
Inflammation (e.g. Kawasaki's disease)
Mailgnancy (e.g. Hodgkin's disease)
Splenectomy
Trauma/surgery

Primary
Essential thrombocythaemia
Polycythaemia vera
Myelofibrosis (initially, later thrombocytopenia)
Myelodysplasia
CML

Pleural effusion
Exudate
Infection: TB, bacterial pneumonia
Inflammation/connective tissue disease, e.g. SLE, sarcoidosis
Malignancy: bronchial carcinoma, mesothelioma
Pulmonary infarction
Post-MI
Pancreatitis (acute)

Transudate
Cardiac failure
Hypoproteinaemia
Hypothyroidism
Constrictive pericarditis
Meigs' syndrome

Pleuritic chest pain
See Chest pain

Poikilocytosis
Iron deficiency anaemia
Thalassaemia
Myelofibrosis

Polydipsia
See Polyuria

Polyarthralgia
Infection: disseminated septic arthritis (e.g. staphylococcal, gonococcal), viral
(e.g. enteroviruses, EBV, HIV, Hepatitis B, mumps, rubella), rheumatic fever,
Lyme disease, TB

Gout/pseudogout
Rheumatoid arthritis, osteoarthritis (generalized)
Seronegative arthritis: (**R**eactive/Reiter's, **E**nteropathic (Whipple's, IBD),
Ankylosing spondylitis, **P**soriatic arthritis)
Systemic diseases: SLE, sarcoid, Sjögren's, Behçet's, primary vasculitides,
polymyalgia rheumatica
Other: haemochromatosis, sickle cell, malignancy (hypertrophic pulmonary
osteoarthropathy)

Migratory polyarthralgia
Gonococcal arthritis
Rheumatic fever

Polychromasia
Haemorrhage
Haematinics (ferrous sulphate, B_{12})
Haemolysis, dyserythropoiesis

Polycythaemia
Relative polycythaemia: dehydration (e.g. alcohol, diuretics), Gaisböck's syndrome
True polycythaemia:
$1°$: Polycythaemia rubra vera
$2°$: Appropriate ↑ in erythropoietin: chronic hypoxia, e.g. high altitude,
chronic lung disease, cyanotic heart disease. Inappropriate ↑ in
erythropoietin, e.g. renal cell carcinoma/cysts, hepatoma, cerebellar
haemangioblastoma, fibroids

Polyneuropathy
Infection: HIV, Lyme disease, leprosy, diphtheria
Inflammation: Guillain–Barré syndrome, chronic inflammatory demyelinating
neuropathy, Sjögren's syndrome, sarcoidosis, SLE, vasculitides (e.g.
polyarteritis nodosa)
Tumours: paraneoplastic, paraproteinaemia
Toxic: alcohol, heavy metals (e.g. lead), insecticides, drugs (cisplatinum,
vincristine, amiodarone, metronidazole, phenytoin, isoniazid, nitrofurantoin,
gold)
Metabolic: diabetes mellitus, hypothyroidism, B_{12}/thiamine deficiency,
amyloidosis, uraemia
Hereditary: e.g. abetalipoproteinaemia, porphyria, Charcot–Marie–Tooth
syndrome, Refsum's syndrome, lysosomal storage diseases, e.g. Fabry's disease,
Niemann–Pick disease

Polyuria
Diabetes mellitus (uncontrolled)
Diabetes insipidus:
Central: tumour, trauma/surgery, infiltration (e.g. TB, sarcoid, histiocytosis X,
lymphocytic hypophysitis, DIDMOAD*)
Nephrogenic: hypercalcaemia, hypokalaemia, Lithium, X-linked)
Diuretics
Diuretic phase of acute renal failure, chronic renal failure
Post-obstructive diuresis
Psychogenic polydypsia

Portal hypertension
Prehepatic: portal/splenic vein thrombosis
Hepatic: cirrhosis, granulomata, schistosomiasis
Posthepatic: Budd–Chiari syndrome (hepatic vein thrombosis), congestive cardiac
  failure, constrictive pericarditis

PR interval
Long
First-degree atrioventricular (AV) block

Short
Wolff–Parkinson–White sndrome
Lown–Ganong–Levine syndrome
Hypertrophic obstructive cardiomyopathy, Duchenne's muscular dystrophy

Priapism
Low flow:
  After normal intercourse
  After self-injection of alprostadil or papaverine for impotence
  α-Blocking agents, e.g. prazosin
  Haematological diseases: sickle cell diseases, leukaemia
  Haemodialysis
High flow (rare):
  Caused by an injury resulting in an aneurysm of the deep artery of the corpus
    cavernosum

Proptosis
Unilateral
Orbital tumour (e.g. optic nerve tumour, Hodgkin's lymphoma, etc.),
  granuloma
Orbital cellulitis

Bilateral
Caroticocavernous fistula
Cavernous sinus thrombosis
Thyrotoxicosis
Orbital abnormalities (craniostenoses: Crouzon or Apert syndrome)

Prostate-specific antigen (PSA)
See Tumour markers

Proteinuria
Pregnancy
Diabetes mellitus
Hypertension
Infection (UTI)
Inflammation (SLE, glomerulonephritis)
Multiple myeloma
Amyloidosis
Other: fever, exercise, CCF, orthostatic proteinuria, contamination (semen,
  vaginal discharge)

Prothrombin time (PT), ↑
Warfarin/vitamin K deficiency
Liver disease

DIC

Heparin

Note: PT monitors the extrinsic pathway i.e. deficiency or inhibition of coagulation factors: VII, X, V, II, fibrinogen

Proximal muscle weakness

Toxic/metabolic: steroids, Cushing's syndrome, thyrotoxicosis, hypothyroidism, osteomalacia

Inflammatory: dermatomyositis, polymyositis, polymyalgia rheumatica

Infection: staphylococcal myositis, parasites (trichinosis, cysticercosis), viral (influenza, coxsackie, echo)

Inherited: muscular dystrophies, metabolic myopathies (e.g. glycogen storage diseases e.g. McArdle's syndrome), mitochondrial myopathies, familial periodic paralysis (associated with hypo/hyperkalaemia)

Pruritus

Cutaneous diseases

Eczema, allergic reactions

Lichen planus

Scabies

Herpes simplex, herpes zoster, parasites

Dermatitis herpetiformis

Blistering disorders

Psoriasis (occasionally)

Nodular prurigo (following insect bites)

Systemic diseases

Metabolic: liver failure, chronic renal failure

Endocrine: hyperthyroidism, hypothyroidism, diabetes mellitus

Haematological: polycythaemia, iron deficiency anaemia, Hodgkin's lymphoma

Psychological: parasitophobia, anxiety

Tropical infection: filariasis, hookworm

Drugs: alkaloids

Pruritus ani

Incontinence, diarrhoea, poor hygiene

Infection: *Enterobius vermicularis* (threadworm), fungal (candidiasis, tinea cruris), scabies

Anal disease: haemorrhoids, fissure, fistula, wart

Skin disease: contact dermatitis, eczema, psoriasis, lichen sclerosis

Other: anxiety, tight pants

Pseudobulbar palsy

See Bulbar palsy

Pseudohermaphrodite

Female

Excess androgens:

↑ Exposure during the embryonic period: androgen from adrenal/ovarian tumour or luteoma of pregnancy, congenital adrenal hyperplasia (CAH), intake of androgens or androgenic progestogens taken by the mother

↑ Synthesis in the adrenals: CAH

Male

Leydig cell hypoplasia

Pseudohermaphrodite continued

Luteinizing hormone (LH) or LH-receptor mutation (autosomal recessive)
Testosterone synthesis defects (autosomal recessive)
5-alpha reductase deficiency (autosomal recessive)
Androgen insensitivity: spectrum varies from partial (Reifenstein's syndrome) →
   complete (testicular feminization syndrome)

Ptosis

Third nerve palsy (*See* Cranial nerve palsy)
Horner's syndrome (*See* Horner's syndrome)
Myopathy:
   Myasthenia gravis
   Myotonic dystrophy
   Ocular myopathy
Congenital
Syphilis

PT

See Prothrombin time

PTT

See APTT

Puberty

Delayed

Constitutional growth and puberty delay
Hypogonadism of pre-pubertal onset (*See* Hypogonadism)

Precocious
Complete (central)

Congenital: hydrocephalus, brain malformations
Acquired: tumours (hypothalamic/pituitary: glioma, hamartomas), trauma,
   radiation, infiltrations

Incomplete
Premature pubic/axillary hair development: excess androgens

Leydig cells stimulated by hCG (which has LH-like activity), e.g. from hepatoma,
   hepatoblastoma, pineal/hypothalamic teratomas
Leydig cells premature activation (testotoxicosis) due to an activating mutation of
   the LH receptor
Leydig cell tumour
McCune–Albright syndrome: constitutive activation of the gonadotrophin
   receptor on Leydig cells
Excess androgens from adrenal tumours, CAH
Exogenous sex steroids

Premature breast development (thelrache): excess oestrogens:

Ovarian cyst (developed possibly due to premature FSH secretion)
Hypothyroidism (↓ thyroid hormone → ↑ TSH stimulates FSH secretion:
   ↑ FSH → ovarian cyst development)
Ovarian neoplasm
McCune–Albright

Pulmonary function tests

See Lung function tests

Pulmonary hypertention

Primary
Secondary:
   Left heart disease (mitral valve disease, LVF, left atrial myxoma/thrombosis)
   Chronic lung disease (COPD)
   Recurrent pulmonary emboli
   ↑ Pulmonary blood flow (VSD, ASD, patent ductus arteriosus)
   Connective tissue disease (e.g. SLE, scleroderma)
   Drugs: fenfluramine (appetite suppressant)
   HIV

Pulse

Tachycardia: *See* Tachycardia
Bradycardia: *See* Bradycardia

Irregular pulse

Sinus arrhythmia (rate increases with inspiration)
Irregularly irregular: atrial fibrillation, multiple ectopic beats (extrasystoles),
   atrial flutter with variable block
Regularly irregular: $2°$ heart block, ventricular bigemini

Bounding pulse

Peripheral vasodilatation: CO_2 retention (e.g. COPD), sepsis, liver failure,
   thyrotoxicosis
↑ Stroke volume: aortic regurgitation, patent ductus arteriosus, large AV fistulas,
   thyrotoxicosis, severe anaemia, exercise

Unequal/delayed pulses

Atherosclerosis, thromboembolic disease
Aortic dissection
Aortic aneurysm
Arteritis: Large vessel vasculitis (Takayasu's arteritis, giant cell arteritis, secondary
   syphilis)
Subclavian steal syndrome
Supravalvular aortic stenosis

Pulse pressure

↑
Aortic regurgitation
Thyrotoxicosis
Pregnancy
Patent ductus arteriosus
High-output cardiac failure (e.g. severe anaemia, beri beri, Paget's disease)

↓
Aortic stenosis
Shock
Pericardial effusion, constrictive pericarditis

Pulsus paradoxicus

Cardiac tamponade, constrictive pericarditis
Asthma (severe)

Pupils

Dilated: *See* Mydriasis
Constricted: *See* Miosis
Unequal: *See* Anisocoria

Purpura

Senile
Steroids (iatrogenic, Cushing's syndrome)
Infection: meningococcal septicaemia/DIC, infective endocarditis
Platelet disorders: quantitative (thrombocytopenia), qualitative (von Willebrand's
   disease), coagulopathy (haemophilia, liver disease, anticoagulants)
Vasculitis: e.g:
   1°: Henoch–Schönlein purpura, polyarteritis nodosa, Churg–Strauss, Wegener's
      granulomatosis, cryoglobulinaemia
   2°: SLE, rheumatoid arthritis
Collagen diseases: scurvy, Ehlers–Danlos syndrome
Others: emboli (e.g. cholesterol), hereditary haemorrhagic telangiectasia,
   amyloidosis

Pustules

Infection:
   Bacterial: Staphylococcal, Gram –ve bacilli, Gonococcal, secondary syphilis
   Viral: HSV, VZV (pustules preceded by vesicles)
   Fungal: (dermatophyte infection inappropriately treated with topical steroids)
   Scabies
Psoriasis (pustular)
Pyoderma gangrenosum
Drugs: steroids, phenytoin, isoniazid
Developing at sites of trauma (pathergy): Behçet's disease, Sweet's syndrome
With other skin signs: acne, rosacea

Pyoderma gangrenosum

Inflammatory bowel disease, autoimmune hepatitis
Rheumatoid arthritis, seronegative arthritides
Haematological: leukaemia, myeloma, polycythaemia rubra vera
Wegener's granulomatosis
Idiopathic (50%)

Pyrexia of unknown origin (PUO)

Infection: abscesses (subphrenic, liver, pelvis)
   Bacterial: infective endocarditis, osteomyelitis, UTI, biliary infection
   TB, brucellosis, viral infections (HIV, CMV, EBV), malaria
Inflammation/CTD: rheumatoid arthritis, SLE, sarcoidosis, vasculitides,
   polymyalgia rheumatica
Malignancy: lymphomas, leukaemia, renal cell carcinoma, hepatocellular
   carcinoma, pancreatic carcinoma
Drugs: e.g. sulphonamides, isoniazid, aspirin
Familial Mediterranean fever (FMF), familial periodic fever (FPF)

Pyuria, sterile

TB, inadequately treated UTI, UTI with fastidious culture requirement
Bladder: tumour, chemical cystitis (e.g. cytotoxics)
Calculi
Renal papillary necrosis (e.g. analgesic excess), interstitial nephritis, polycystic
   kidney disease
Prostatitis
Appendicitis

Q

Q waves

Normal
   If < 25% of the height of the following R wave or < 2 mm deep
   'Septal' Q waves in the lateral leads
   Common in III, V_5-V_6
Myocardial infarction (> a few hours' duration)
Left ventricular hypertrophy
Bundle branch block

QRS complexes

Axis deviation: *See* Axis deviation
Bundle branch block: *See* Bundle branch blocks
Low voltage QRS complexes
   Incorrect standardization
   Obesity
   COPD
   Pericardial effusion
   Myxoedema
Wide QRS complexes
   Ventricular extrasystoles, ventricular tachycardia, complete AV block
   Bundle branch block: Left and Right
   Left anterior hemiblock
Dominant R waves in V_1: *See* R wave

QT interval

Long

Hypothermia
Hypocalcaemia, hypokalaemia, hypomagnesaemia
Congenital: Romano–Ward syndrome, Jervell–Lange–Nielsen syndrome
Drugs: tricyclic antidepressants, chloroquine, Class Ia anti-arrhythmic drugs
Acute MI, acute myocarditis
Cerebral injury

Short

Hyperthermia
Hypercalcaemia
Digoxin

R

R wave, dominant in V1
Right ventricular hypertrophy, right BBB, pulmonary embolism
Posterior MI
Myocarditis
Wolff–Parkinson–White syndrome (left-sided accessory pathway)
Misplaced pacemaker! (in left atrium)

Rash
Cutaneous diseases, e.g. eczema, psoriasis, urticaria
Drugs
Infection (bacterial, viral, fungal, parasitic)
Inflammatory/connective tissue diseases
Malignancy
See also Hyperpigmentation, Hypopigmented macules, Photodistributed rash

Raynaud's phenomenon
Idiopathic
Occupational (vibrating tools)
Connective tissue diseases: scleroderma, SLE, Sjögren's syndrome, rheumatoid
    arthritis, dermatomyositis
Cold agglutinins
Cryoglobulinaemia, macroglobulinaemia (Waldenström's)
Cervical rib
Drugs: β-blockers
Vascular disease

Rectal discharge
Common
Haemorrhoids
Anal fissure
Rectal prolapse
Proctitis
Perianal warts

Occasional
Rectal carcinoma
Anal fistula
Perianal IBD
Solitary rectal ulcer syndrome
Villous adenoma

Rarely
Infection: anal TB, gonorrhoea, syphilis, HIV
Anal carcinoma

Red blood cell fragmentation
Artificial heart valve/artificial graft
Microangiopathic haemolytic anaemia
    DIC, HUS, TTP, malignant hypertension, meningococcal septicaemia,
    pre-eclampsia
    Widespread adenocarcinoma

Red eye
Conjunctivitis (allergic, viral, bacterial, chlamydial)
Episcleritis
Scleritis
Iritis (anterior uveitis)
Acute angle closure glaucoma
Other: inflamed pinguecula, subconjuctival haemorrhage
See also Painful red eye

Red reflex, absent
Cataract
Corneal oedema (acute angle closure glaucoma)
Vitreous hemorrhage
Retinal detachment

Reflexes
Reflexes
  ↑: *See* Upper motor neurone lesion
  ↓: *See* Lower motor neurone lesion

Absent reflexes with up–going plantars
Motor neurone disease
Friedreich's ataxia
Subacute combined degeneration of the cord (B_{12} deficiency)
Spinal shock
Tabes dosalis
Pellagra
Conus medullaris lesion
Severe hyponatraemia

Relative afferent pupillary defect (RAPD)
Optic neuritis
Optic nerve compression
Central retinal artery occlusion
Retinal detachment
Glaucoma (unilateral)

Renal tubular acidosis
Type 1
Autoimmune: Sjögren's syndrome, SLE, primary biliary cirrhosis
Nephrocalcinosis: hypercalcaemia, medullary sponge kidney
Obstructive uropathy
Toxic: amphotericin, Lithium, transplanted kidney (rejection)
Sickle cell anaemia
(Mnemonic: **A**cid **NOT** **S**ecreted)

Type 2
Acquired: myeloma, hyperparathyroidism, vitamin D deficiency, Drugs:
  acetazolamide, heavy metals
Congenital: as part of Fanconi's syndrome, fructose intolerance, cystinosis,
  Wilson's disease, tyrosinaemia

Type 4
Diabetes mellitus
Pyelonephritis

Renal tubular acidosis continued
Drugs: NSAIDs, potassium-sparing diuretics
Urinary obstruction
Sickle cell disease

Respiratory failure
Type 1: *See* Arterial blood gas
Type 2: *See* Arterial blood gas

Respiratory rate
↑
Physiological: exercise, anxiety
Lung disease: pneumothorax, pulmonary embolism, obstructive disease, e.g.
   asthma attack, restrictive disease, infection, inflammation (vasculitis),
   malignancy
Elevation of diaphragm: ascites, diaphragmatic paralysis
Metabolic acidosis

↓
Physiological: well-conditioned athletes
CNS disease: infection (meningitis, encephalitis), trauma (head injury), tumour
   (↑ intracranial pressure), drugs (sedatives), coma

Reticulocytosis
Haemolysis
Haemorrhage
After the response to B_{12}/folate/iron treatment given to marrow that lack these

Retinal haemorrhages
Central retinal vein occlusion
Diabetic retinopathy
Hypertension
Papillloedema

Retinal neovascularization
Diabetic proliferative retinopathy
Retinal vein thrombosis
Sickle cell haemoglobinopathy
SLE
Ocular ischaemic syndrome (due to carotid occlusive disease)
Eales disease (peripheral retinal vasculitis)

Retinitis pigmentosa
Abetalipoproteinaemia
Laurence–Moon–Biedl
Refsum's disease
Friedreich's ataxia and other hereditary ataxias
Familial neuropathies
Neuronal lipidoses (ceroid lipofuscinosis)

Rheumatoid factor, +ve
Sjögren's syndrome (95%)
Rheumatoid arthritis (70%)
SLE
Scleroderma

Mixed connective tissue disease
Mixed cryoglobulinaemia
Polymyositis/dermatomyositis
Infection/inflammatory diseases, e.g. TB, infectious mononucleosis, subacute
    bacterial endocarditis, chronic hepatitis
Healthy individuals (~5%)

Rigors
Cholangitis
Pyelonephritis
Pneumococcal pneumonia
Malaria
Localized sepsis (abscesses)

Roth's spots
Infective endocarditis
Leukaemia
Anaemia
Vasculitis: PAN, SLE

Rubeosis iris
Proliferative retinopathy (diabetes mellitus, sickle cell disease, retinal vein
    thrombosis)
Carotid artery disease including carotid–cavernous fistula
Chronic intraocular inflammation/tumour
Chronic retinal detachment

S

Saddle nose deformity
Trauma
Congenital syphilis
Wegener's granulomatosis
Relapsing polychondritis
Lepromatous leprosy

Scleromalacia perforans
Rheumatoid arthritis
Ankylosing spondylitis
Vasculitis (Wegener's granulomatosis, polyarteritis nodosa)
Gout
Herpes zoster

Scotoma, central
Optic nerve disease
Retinal disease affecting the macula

Scrotal swelling
See Masses and swellings

Seizures
Adults
Vascular: infarction, haemorrhage, cortical venous thrombosis, vascular
    malformation
Trauma: head injury
Tumours
Toxic: alcohol, drugs, lead, carbon monoxide
Metabolic: hypoxia, hypoglycaemia, electrolyte disturbances ($\uparrow$ or $\downarrow$ Na$^+$, K$^+$, Ca^{2+},
    Mg^{2+}), renal/hepatic failure, endocrine disorders (hypopituitarism,
    myxoedema, hypo/hyperparathyroidism, Addison's disease, insulinoma),
    vitamin deficiency
Infection: meningitis, encephalitis, abscess, TB, cysticercosis, HIV
Inflammation: MS, vasculitis, SLE, sarcoidosis
Degenerative disorders: Alzheimer's disease, prion disease
Very raised BP

Children
Congenital anomaly
Tuberous sclerosis
Metabolic storage diseases

Sensory disturbance, distribution
Hemisensory loss (arm, trunk, leg) + ipsilateral facial sensory loss:
    Contralateral thalamic lesion
Hemisensory + contralateral facial sensory loss:
    Contralateral brainstem (ipsilateral to the facial sensory loss)
Bilateral lower limbs and trunk (below a dermatomal sensory level):
    $\downarrow$*Pin prick/temperature sensation:* bilateral spinothalamic tracts
    $\downarrow$*Joint position/vibration sensation:* bilateral dorsal columns

Hemisensory loss (leg and trunk below a dermatomal sensory level):
  ↓ *Pin prick/temperature sensation:* contralateral spinothalamic tracts
  ↓ *Joint position/vibration sensation:* ipsilateral dorsal columns
Upper arms and trunk ('suspended sensory loss' for pin prick and temperature):
  Central spinal cord (e.g. syringomyelia)
Glove-and-stocking:
  Peripheral neuropathy
  Cervical myelopathy
Dermatomal
Peripheral nerve

Sensory disturbance, timing of onset
Transient
Epilepsy
Migraine
TIA, stroke
CNS demyelination
Peripheral nerve or root entrapment
Psychogenic

Persistent
Brain: space-occupying lesions (tumour, subdural haematoma, abscess)
Spinal cord: cervical spondylosis, demyelination
Nerve root: spondylitic radiculopathy
Peripheral nerve: peripheral neuropathy e.g. diabetes mellitus (*See*
  Polyneuropathy)

SGOT
See Liver function tests

SGPT
See Liver function tests

Short 4th/5th finger
Turner's syndrome
Pseudohypoparathyroidism
Dactylitis residua (sickle cell disease)

Shortness of breath
See under Breathlessness

Shoulder pain
Overuse injuries, subluxation, fracture
Adhesive capsulitis (frozen shoulder)
Rotator cuff tendinitis
Subacromial bursitis
Rotator cuff tear
Bicipital tendinitis
Arthritis (septic, osteoarthritis, rheumatoid arthritis, gout/pseudogout)
Acute calcific tendinitis
Avascular necrosis
Referred pain:
  Myocardial ischaemia (left shoulder pain)
  Cervical disc herniation/spinal stenosis, nerve entrapment (long thoracic or
    suprascapular nerve)

Shoulder pain continued
Diaphragmatic irritation (e.g. subphrenic abscess), hepatic capsule distension, pulmonary tumour/infection/abscess

Skin necrosis
Warfarin, Protein C/S deficiency, DIC (e.g. meningococcal septicaemia)
Vasculitis (Primary: Wegener's granulomatosis, cryoglobulinaemia; Secondary: SLE, rheumatoid arthritis)
Peripheral vascular disease
Emboli: cholesterol, subacute bacterial endocarditis
Pyoderma gangrenosum
Panniculitis (e.g. idiopathic, pancreatitis)
Calciphylaxis (small-vessel vasculitis causing skin necrosis associated with end-stage renal failure, $\uparrow Ca^{2+}$ and phosphate)

Snoring
Obstructive sleep apnoea
Airway narrowing:
  Low-set thick soft palate, longer-than-normal uvula
  Tongue falling backwards when sleeping supine
  Enlarged tonsils, nasal blockage (e.g. allergies, deviated septum)
$\uparrow$ Upper-airway soft-tissue laxity and muscle weakness:
  $\uparrow$ Age, obesity, alcohol/tranquilizers

Sore throat
Pharyngitis (viral)
Streptococcal tonsillitis
Infectious mononucleosis
Gonococcal pharyngitis
Diphtheria

With pharyngeal ulcers
Herpes simplex
Herpangina
Vincent's angina (fusospirochetal infection)
Candidiasis

Spastic paraparesis
Cord compression (cervical spondylosis, disc prolapse, secondary tumour in spine, spinal cord tumour)
Multiple sclerosis
Motor neurone disease
Trauma, birth injury (cerebral palsy)
Syringomyelia

Others
Vascular: anterior spinal artery thrombosis, venous sinus thrombosis, multiple cerebral infarctions
Infection: tranverse myelitis (post-infectious, e.g. Mycoplasma), HIV, HTLV-1 (tropical spastic paraparesis), syphilis
Tumours: parasigittal meningioma
Toxic/metabolic: B_{12} deficiency (subacute combined degeneration)
Congenital: hereditary spastic paraparesis, Friedreich's ataxia

Spherocytosis
Hereditary spherocytosis
Autoimmune haemolytic anaemia
Septicaemia

Splenomegaly
Massive
Chronic myeloid leukaemia, myelofibrosis
Tropical infections: malaria, leishmaniasis, schistosomiasis, tropical splenomegaly
Gaucher's disease

Moderate
Haematological (haemolytic anaemia, lymphoma, leukaemia, myeloproliferative disorders*)
Portal hypertension (See Portal hypertension)
Infection: infective endocarditis, infectious mononucleosis, tuberculosis, brucellosis
Inflammatory/connective tissue diseases: rheumatoid arthritis, SLE, sarcoidosis, amyloidosis

*Chronic myeloid leukaemia, myelofibrosis, polycythaemia rubra vera, essential thrombocythaemia.

Splinter haemorrhages
Trauma, e.g. gardening
Infective endocarditis
Vasculitis
Psoriasis
Mitral stenosis

Sputum (purulent)
Upper respiratory source (acute sinusitis, rhinitis, bronchitis)
Infection: pneumonia, TB, lung abscess
Bronchiectasis
Bronchopleural fistula
See also Haemoptysis

ST segment
Depression
Myocardial ischaemia
Myocardial infarction (posterior)
Drugs (digoxin, quinidine)
Ventricular hypertrophy

Elevation
Myocardial infarction (acute)
Pericarditis
Prinzmetal angina
Left ventricular aneurysm
High take-off

Stature
Short stature
CGPD (constitutional growth and puberty delay), familial
Syndromic: Turner's syndrome, achondroplasia, Prader–Willi

Stature continued

Psychosocial factors: child abuse, anorexia nervosa, emotional deprivation
Endocrine factors:
  ↓ Growth hormone: Hypopituitarism (e.g. pituitary tumour)
  Mutations: Pit1, PROP1, GHRH receptor
  Cushing's syndrome and ↑↑ corticosteroids
  Biologically inactive GH
  GH resistance (GH-receptor mutation)
  Low levels of IGF1 (Laron dwarfism)
  ↓ Thyroid hormones (hypothyroidism)
Nutritional factors
Systemic illness:
  Gastrointestinal: malabsorption (coeliac disease, milk protein intolerance,
    inflammatory bowel disease)
  Cardiovascular: congenital cyanotic heart disease
  Respiratory: cystic fibrosis
  Renal: chronic renal failure

Tall stature

Familial
Syndromic (disproportionate):
  Klinefelter's syndrome
  Marfan's syndrome
  Homocystinuria
Endocrine:
  Excess GH (gigantism)
  Excess thyroid hormones (thyrotoxicosis)
  Excess sex steroids/precocious puberty (e.g. early phases of CAH, adrenal
    tumours)

Steatorrhoea
Small bowel disease/resection

Bacterial overgrowth (e.g. scleroderma, diverticulosis, autonomic neuropathy),
  coeliac disease, Crohn's disease, ileocaecal TB, parasite infection (e.g.
  giardiasis, strongyloidiasis), intestinal lymphoma, radiation enteritis,
  Whipple's disease, tropical sprue

Pancreatic insufficiency

Chronic pancreatitis, pancreatic cancer, cystic fibrosis

Biliary insufficiency

Biliary obstruction, primary biliary cirrhosis

Striae

Cushing's syndrome
Systemic steroids
Physiological: pregnancy (lower abdomen, breasts), adolescence (thighs,
  lumbosacral areas), weight-lifters (shoulders)

Stridor

Partial obstruction of upper airways
Intraluminal:
  Foreign body, tumour

Intramural:
  Infection: epiglottitis, croup in children, respiratory papillomata (HPV warts on
    the larynx), retropharyngeal abscess
  Laryngeal oedema (anaphylaxis, smoke inhalation)
  Laryngeal carcinoma
  Cricoarytenoid rheumatoid arthritis
  Tracheal stenosis (following surgery/intubation/tracheostomy)
Extramural:
  Goitre
  Lymphadenopathy

Sweating
↑ Sweating: See Hyperhidrosis
See also Night sweats

T

T waves
Tall
Hyperkalaemia
Acute MI
Normal variant

Small
Hypokalaemia
Pericardial effusion
Hypothyroidism

Inverted
V_1—V_3/V_4
Normal variant (children and black people)
Right bundle branch block
Pulmonary embolism

V_2—V_5
Non-Q wave MI
Hypertrophic cardiomyopathy
Subarachnoid haemorrhage, Lithium

V_4—V_6 and lateral
Left ventricular hypertrophy
Myocardial ischaemia
Associated with LBBB

Tachycardia
Sinus tachycardia
Fever, exercise, anxiety, anaemia, drugs (caffeine, salbutamol, anticholinergics, catecholamines, nicotine), pregnancy
Hypotension (e.g. hypovolaemia, septicaemia)
Cardiac: MI, congestive cardiac failure, constrictive pericarditis
Pulmonary: pulmonary embolism, asthma, chronic lung disease
Endocrine: hyperthyroidism, phaeochromocytomas, hypoglycaemia

Supraventricular tachycardia
Idiopathic, Wolff–Parkinson–White syndrome

Atrial fibrillation/flutter
Idiopathic, thyrotoxicosis, alcohol abuse, pulmonary: embolism/infection/cancer, pericarditis, cardiomyopathy, ischaemic heart disease, rheumatic heart disease, mitral stenosis

Ventricular tachycardia
Idiopathic, ischaemic heart disease/MI, hypertensive heart disease, cardiomyopathy, myocarditis, long QT syndrome, drugs

Tachypnoea
See Respiratory rate

Target cells
Splenectomy
Haemoglobinopathies (sickle cell anaemia, thalassaemia, haemoglobin C disease)
Iron deficiency
Liver disease
Lecithin cholesterol acyltransferase (LCAT) deficiency

Taste impairment
See under Dysgeusia

Teardrop cells
Thalassaemia
Bone marrow fibrosis

Telangiectasia
Normal variant
Connective tissue diseases: scleroderma, SLE, dermatomyositis
Genetic: hereditary haemorrhagic telangiectasia, ataxia telangiectasia
Chronic liver disease (esp. alcoholic cirrhosis)
Pregnancy
Topical steroids (long-term)
Rosacea
Radiation dermatitis

Tenesmus
Space-occupying lesions in rectal wall/lumen, e.g. rectal carcinoma
Irritable bowel syndrome

Testicular atrophy
See Hypogonadism, male

Testicular pain and swelling
Testicular torsion
Epidydimo-orchitis
TB, sarcoid
Leukaemia
Polyarteritis nodosa, Henoch–Schönlein
Renal vein thrombosis

Testosterone, ↓
See Hypogonadism

Thrombin time, ↑
DIC (↓ fibrinogen)
Heparin

Thrombocytopenia
See Platelets

Thrombocytosis
See Platelets

Thyroid-binding globulin (TBG)
↑ levels
Genetic

Thyroid-binding globulin (TBG) continued
Pregnancy
Drugs (oestrogen, opiates, phenothiazines)
Acute viral hepatitis, acute intermittent porphyria

↓ **levels**
Genetic
Malnutrition
Chronic liver disease
Nephrotic syndrome
Drugs (e.g. androgens, corticosteroids)
Acromegaly

Thyroid function tests
Normal T4, T3 and TSH: Euthyroid
Normal T4 and T3, ↓ TSH: Sub-clinical hyperthyroidism, same causes as overt
   hyperthyroidism
Normal T4 and T3, ↑ TSH: Subclinical hypothyroidism, same causes as overt
   hypothyroidism
↓ T4 and T3, ↑ TSH: Primary hypothyroidism (See Hypothyroidism)
↓ T4 and T3, ↓ or normal TSH: Secondary hypothyroidism (See Hypopituitarism),
   sick euthyroid syndrome (systemic illness, esp. hospitalized patients)
↑ T4 and T3, ↓ TSH: Primary hyperthyroidism (See Hyperthyroidism)
↑ T4 and T3, normal or ↑ TSH: Secondary hyperthyroidism (pituitary TSHoma),
   resistance to thyroid hormone
↑ T4 and T3, normal TSH: ↑ Serum thyroxine-binding globulin
   Familial dysalbuminaemic hyperthyroxinaemia
   Anti-T4 antibodies

Tingling in hands and feet
See Paraesthesia

Tinnitus
Local
Presbycusis
Ménière's disease
Noise-induced
Ototoxic drugs, e.g. aminoglycosides, loop diuretics
Otosclerosis
Aneursms/AV malformations
Tumours: acoustic neuroma, glomus jugulare tumour, carotid body tumour
Temporomandibular joint problems
Insects, e.g. maggots

General
Fever
CVS: hypertension, heart failure
Haematological: ↑ viscosity, anaemia
CNS: multiple sclerosis
Drugs: aspirin, alcohol, quinine

Tongue
Furring
Smokers

Mouth breathers
Drugs, e.g. antibiotics
Dehydration
GI diseases

Sore tongue
Ulcers: infection (herpes simplex), inflammatory (Behçet's disease), malignancy
Glossitis (iron/folate/vitamin B/riboflavin deficiency, candidiasis) See Glossitis
Sore physiologically normal tongue
Psychogenic
Swelling (See Macroglossia)
Ulceration
Aphthous ulcer
Dental trauma
Tumour
Syphilis

Tracheal deviation
Collapse
Tension pneumothorax
Large pleural effusion

Transfer factor
See Lung function tests

Tremor
Essential tremor: (postural tremor of hands/head, e.g. when holding a glass/
writing, positive family history, ↓ with alcohol or β-blockers)
Physiological tremor: (made worse by hyperthyroidism, anxiety, alcohol, drugs,
e.g. β-agonist bronchodilators, valproate, lithium, antidepressants)
Tremor at rest: Parkinson's disease and other akinetic–rigid syndromes
Action tremor: cerebellar sign (See Cerebellar signs)

Tricuspid regurgitation
Congenital: Ebstein's anomaly (malpositioned tricuspid valve), cleft tricuspid
valve in ostium primum ASD
Infective endocarditis (common in IV drug users)
Rheumatic heart disease (associated with tricuspid stenosis or other vavular
disease)
Carcinoid syndrome, cirrhosis (long-standing), Drugs: fenfluramine,
methysergide, endomyocardial fibrosis (may be associated with
hypereosinophilia)
Functional: consequence of right ventricular dilatation (e.g. in pulmonary
hypertension, myocardial infarction), valve prolapse (e.g. in Marfan's
syndrome)
Iatrogenic: radiotherapy to the thorax, TR seen after a successful mitral valvotomy
for mitral stenosis

Troponin T, ↑
Myocardial infarction
May also be elevated in: unstable angina, chronic renal failure

Tumour markers, ↑
α-Fetoprotein: hepatoma, germ-cell tumour, pregnancy, hepatitis, cirrhosis,
open neural tube defects

Tumour markers, ↑ continued

CA 125: ovarian cancer, other malignancies (breast, endometrial, lung, pancreas). Benign conditions (endometriosis, fibroids, pelvic inflammatory disease, peritonitis, cirrhosis)

CA 15–3: breast cancer, benign breast disease

CA 19–9: pancreatic cancer, colorectal cancer, cholestasis

CEA: colorectal cancer, medullary thyroid carcinoma, cirrhosis, pancreatitis, smoking

HCG: pregnancy, germ cell tumours, hydatidiform mole, choriocarcinoma

PLAP: seminoma, smoking, pregnancy, ovarian carcinoma

PSA: prostate cancer, benign prostatic hyperplasia, prostatitis, digital rectal examination, (PSA also ↑ with age and size of the gland)

Tunnel vision

Retinitis pigmentosa (*See* Retinitis pigmentosa)

Chronic glaucoma

Chronic papilloedema

U

U wave
Normal
Hypokalaemia
Hypercalcaemia
Hyperthyroidism

Ulcers: mouth, genital, leg
Mouth
Trauma, aphthous ulcers
Gastrointestinal diseases: Crohn's disease, coeliac disease
Infection: herpes simplex, acute ulcerative stomatitis (Vincent's angina),
    candidiasis TB, syphilis (rare)
    Exclude: leukaemia, agranulocytosis
Inflammatory: Behçet's disease, reactive arthritis, SLE
Skin diseases: pemphigus, pemphigoid, erythema multiforme, lichen planus
Malignancy: squamous cell carcinoma
Other: Strachan's syndrome

Genital
Infection: Painful: herpes simplex, *Haemophilus ducreyi* (chancroid)
    Painless: Syphilis (*Treponema pallidum*), Lymphogranuloma venereum
    (*Chlamydia trachomatis*), Granuloma inguinale (*Calymmatobacterium
    granulomatis*)
Behçet's disease
Crohn's disease
Reiter's syndrome
Erythroplasia of Queyrat, squamous cell carcinoma
Trauma
Other genital rashes: fixed drug eruption, eczema, psoriasis, scabies

Orogenital
Infection: herpes simplex, syphilis
Inflammatory diseases: Behçet's disease, Reiter's syndrome
Skin diseases: pemphigus, erythema multiforme
GI: Crohn's disease
Other: Strachan's diseases

Leg
Venous: superficial venous insufficiency, DVT
Arterial: atherosclerosis
Diabetic: ischaemic and neuropathic
Vasculitis: rheumatoid arthritis, primary vasculities, e.g. polyarteritis nodosa
Sickle cell anaemia
Pressure
Pyoderma gangrenosum
Malignancy

Upper motor neurone lesions
See Hemiparesis and Spastic paraparesis

Urea (↑ and ↓)

↑
Impaired glomerular filtration rate (GFR)
High protein diet, GI haemorrhage, catabolic states
Dehydration
Drugs: steroids, tetracycline

↓
Increased GFR (pregnancy)
Low-protein diet, starvation, liver failure
SIADH
Drugs: sodium valproate

Urethral discharge
See Genital discharge

Urgency
UTI
Bladder: stone, tumour, compression by pelvic mass
Prostate enlargement (BPH, cancer)
Genuine stress incontinence, detrusor instability, sensory urgency

Urinalysis
Urine colour
Red/brown
Haematuria
Haemoglobinuria
Myoglobinuria
Beetroot
Porphyria
Phenazopyridine

Rare
White: pyuria, phosphate crystals
Green: methylene blue, amitryptiline, propofol
Dark: obstructive jaundice, ochronosis, malignancy
Orange: rifampicin

Protein
See Proteinuria

Blood
See Haematuria

Urine glucose
See Glycosuria

Ketones
See Ketonuria

Urine leukocyte esterase
Urinary tract infection
Vaginal contaminant

Urine nitrite
Urinary tract infection
Gross haematuria

Urine specific gravity
↑
Dehydration (e.g. diarrhoea, vomiting)
Diabetes mellitus
Adrenal insufficiency
Heart failure
Liver disease
X-ray contrast

↓
Diabetes insipidus
Excessive hydration
Renal failure

Urinary frequency
See Frequency

Urinary incontinence
Stress incontinence
Females: pelvic floor weakness/bladder neck descent (pregnancy, vaginal
    delivery, obesity, menopause)
Males: prostate surgery (external urethral sphincter damage)

Urge incontinence
Detrusor instability (idiopathic, secondary to bladder outflow obstruction, loss of
    supra-spinal inhibition with UMN lesions, e.g. CVA, MS, cord compression: disc
    lesions/spinal tumours, spinal cord/head injury)
Bladder stone, tumour, infection (cystitis)

Continuous incontinence
Chronic retention/overdistension/overflow:
    Outflow obstruction (*see* urinary retention)
    Bladder atonia due to damage to S2, S3, S4 parasympathetic fibres in lower
    spinal cord, cauda equina or pelvis, diabetic autonomic neuropathy
    Fistula (e.g. vesicovaginal) secondary to obstructed labour, surgery,
    malignancy, radiotherapy
Note: Detrusor instability and chronic retention/overdistension of bladder can
    also cause stress incontinence.

Urinary retention, acute
Males
Prostatic hyperplasia/carcinoma
Obstruction of urethral lumen/bladder neck (stricture, stone, tumour, blood clot)
Post-operative*
Medication:, e.g. anticholinergics, antidepressants, alcohol
Neurological: multiple sclerosis, spinal cord disease, e.g. injury/compression,
    diabetic autonomic neuropathy

Females
Pelvic mass: fibroids, ovarian mass, pregnancy (and trauma of labour)
Obstruction of urethral lumen/bladder neck (stone, tumour, blood clot)

Urinary retention, acute continued

Post-operative*

Medication:, e.g. anticholinergics, antidepressants, alcohol

Neurological: multiple sclerosis, spinal cord disease, e.g. injury/compression, diabetic autonomic neuropathy

*Post-operative: drugs/anaesthetics, immobility, constipation, pain, local oedema, neuropraxia, pre-existing bladder outflow obstruction.

Urinary tract obstruction

In the lumen: stones, tumour, blood clots, sloughed renal papillae (NSAIDs, diabetes mellitus, sickle cell)

In the wall: stricture (ureteric/urethral), defective peristalsis, neuropathic bladder

Pressure from the outside: prostatic/pelvic mass, retroperitoneal fibrosis, phimosis

Urine microscopy

Bacteria

Urinary tract infection

Asymptomatic bacteriuria

Contamination

Casts

Epithelial cell casts: acute glomerulonephritis, acute tubular necrosis

Fatty casts: moderate/heavy proteinuria

Granular casts, finely granulated: concentrated urine, diuretics (loop), exercise, fever

Granular casts, densely granulated: glomerulonephritis, interstitial nephritis, diabetic nephropathy, amyloidosis

Hyaline casts: same as finely granulated granular casts

Red cell casts: glomerulonephritis, vasculitis, malignant hypertension

Waxy casts: advanced renal failure

White cell casts: pyelonephritis, proliferative glomerulonephritis

Cells

White cells: UTI (pyelonephritis, cystitis, urethritis), pyuria without bacteriuria: culture inhibited by antibacterial agent or wrong growth condition for fastidious organisms, TB, renal/bladder calculi, glomerulonephritis, interstitial nephritis, analgesic nephropathy, chemical cystitis

Red cells: See Haematuria

Tumour cells: Genitourinary malignancy e.g. bladder cancer, infiltration of renal parenchyma e.g. lymphoma

Crystals

Calcium oxalate (dumbbell-shaped, envelope-shaped, needle-shaped)

Calcium phosphate

Cystine (hexagonal shape)

Magnesium ammonium phosphate (coffin-lid-shaped)

Uric acid (rhombic plates, rosettes)

Uveitis

Inflammatory/Connective tissue diseases: Seronegative spondylarthropathies: (reactive arthritis, enteropathic (inflammatory bowel disease), ankylosing spondylitis, psoriatic arthritis), sarcoidosis, Behçet's desease, juvenile chronic arthritis

Infection: CMV, toxoplasmosis, post-operative infection, fungal, herpetic, TB, syphilis, *Toxocara*

Ocular disease: e.g. sympathetic ophthalmitis, intraocular tumours

V

Vaginal discharge
Physiological: around ovulation, pregnancy, COC pills
Infection
  Candidiasis
  Bacterial vaginosis
  Trichomoniasis
  Chlamydia
  Gonorrhea
  Herpes genitalis
Malignancy (cervical/endometrial)
Foreign body (e.g. retained tampons, swabs)
Other: cervical ectropion, atrophic vaginitis

Vertigo
Labyrinth:
  Acute labyrinthitis
  Benign positional vertigo
  Ménière's disease
  Secondary to middle ear disease
Vestibular nerve:
  Herpes zoster
  Acoustic neuroma
  Ototoxic drugs (e.g. aminoglycosides)
Brainstem:
  Ischaemia (vertebrobasilar circulation)/bleeding
  Multiple sclerosis, tumours
Other:
  Migraine
  Vertiginous epilepsy

Vesicles
See Bullous skin lesions

Visual loss
Sudden
Unilateral
Amaurosis fugax
Central retinal vein occlusion
Central retinal artery occlusion
Vitreous haemorrhage
Retinal detachment
Giant cell arteritis
Optic neuritis

Bilateral
Severe bilateral papilloedema (malignant hypertension, ↑↑ intracranial
  pressure)
Rapid progression of a lesion compressing the optic chiasm
Bilateral infarcts of occipital lobes
Bilateral optic neuritis (rare)

Gradual
Cataracts
Glaucoma
Diabetic retinopathy
Macular degeneration (age-related)
Optic nerve compression

Vomiting

Drugs, poisoning, alcohol
Abdominal pathology (gastrointestinal, hepatic, gynaecological)
Metabolic/endocrine: diabetic ketoacidosis, Addisonian crisis, hypercalcaemia, uraemia, pregnancy
Neurological: increased intracranial pressure (infection, space-occupying lesion, benign intracranial hypertension), acute labyrinthitis
Acute angle closure glaucoma

W

Wasting of small muscles of hands
T1
MND, spinal cord compression, syringomyelia, syphilis, poliomyelitis

Root involvement
Cervical spondylosis, neurofibromata

Brachial plexus involvement
Cervical rib, apical lung tumour, trauma

Peripheral nerve involvement
Rheumatoid arthritis, ulnar/median nerve palsy

Watering eyes
Punctal/lid malposition
Punctal stenosis
Blockage of nasolacrimal duct/Lacrimal sac
↑ Tear production (Can occur paradoxically in patients with dry eyes)

Weak legs
Spastic paraparesis: *See* Spastic paraparesis
Flaccid paraparesis: *See* Flaccid paraparesis
Foot drop: *See* Foot drop

Webbed neck
Turner's syndrome
Klippel–Feil syndrome

Weight loss
Voluntary: diet, exercise

With ↑ appetite
Marked ↑ in physical activity
Malabsorption syndromes
Endocrine: hyperthyroidism, uncontrolled diabetes mellitus,
    phaeochromocytomas

With ↓ appetite
Chronic systemic illness:
    Infections (e.g. TB, brucellosis, subacute bacterial endocarditis, HIV)
    Malignancy
    Cardiopulmonary diseases
    Gastrointestinal disease
    Endocrine diseases, e.g. Addison's disease
Psychiatric: depression, eating disorder (e.g. anorexia nervosa)
Drugs: antidepressants, L-dopa, digoxin, metformin, NSAIDs, alcohol, opiates,
    amphetamine, cocaine

Weight gain
Pregnancy

Excessive caloric intake
Endocrine: PCOS, Cushing's syndrome, hypothyroidism, hypothalamic disease
(trauma, tumour), acromegaly
Drugs: steroids, OCPs, androgenic steroids, antidepressants, anticonvulsants
Depression
↑ Fluid: congestive cardiac failure, renal failure, cirrhosis, excess IV fluids,
lymphatic obstruction
Cessation of cigarette smoking

Wheeze
Narrowing of airways:
Asthma
Bronchitis
Bronchiectasis
Foreign body
Tumour
Left ventricular failure
Carcinoid syndrome
Pulmonary eosinophilia (e.g. tropical eosinophilia, allergic bronchopulmonary
aspergillosis, polyarteritis nodosa)

White cell count
Neutrophils
↑
Infection (bacterial)
Inflammation/connective tissue diseases/vasculitis
Tissue damage: trauma/surgery, burns, MI
Haemorrhage/haemolysis (acute)
Myeloproliferative disease: polycythaemia, chronic myeloid leukaemia
Medication: steroids
Malignancy: particularly disseminated solid tumours and necrotic tumours

↓
As part of a pancytopenia (*See* Pancytopenia)
Infection: viral (e.g. hepatitis, HIV, influenza), typhoid, TB, brucellosis, kala-azar
Drugs: e.g. sulfasalazine, sulphonamides, carbimazole, clozapine
Immune: autoimmune neutropenia, SLE, Felty's syndrome
Benign racial: black Africans
Congenital: Kostmann's syndrome

Eosinophils
↑
Allergic/atopic diseases (asthma, urticaria, eczema, hay fever, food allergy)
Drug sensitivity (e.g. penicillin, sulphonamides)
Parasitic infections (e.g. amoebiasis, ascariasis, *Ankylostoma duodenale*,
schistosomiasis, *Strongyloides stercoralis*, trichinosis, tapeworm,
Toxocara sp.)
Recovery from acute infection
Skin diseases: psoriasis, pemphigus, dermatitis herpetiformis, scabies
Pulmonary eosinophilia (Helminthic infections, allergic bronchopulmonary
aspergillosis, Churg–Strauss syndrome, eosinophilic pneumonia,
hypereosinophilic syndrome)
Polyarteritis nodosa
Addison's disease
Hodgkin's disease and some other tumours, eosinophilic leukaemia

White cell count continued
Lymphocytes
↑

Infections, e.g. viral, toxoplasmosis, TB, brucellosis, pertussis

Chronic lymphocytic leukaemia, prolymphocytic leukaemia, acute lymphoblastic leukaemia, hairy cell leukaemia,

Non-Hodgkin's lymphoma

Thyrotoxicosis

↓

Pancytopenia (e.g. marrow infiltration, chemotherapy/radiation)

Infection: AIDS, legionnaires' disease

Steroids

SLE

Uraemia

Monocytes
↑

Infection: TB, brucellosis, subacute bacterial endocarditis, syphilis, typhoid, viral, e.g. EBV, protozoa

Malignancy: chronic myelomonocytic leukaemia, AML (M4, M5), Hodgkin's disease

Recovery phase of neutropenia

Basophils
↑

Viral infections

Myeloproliferative disorders: polycythaemia rubra vera, chronic myeloid leukaemia

Myxoedema

Ulcerative colitis

Urticaria

Urticaria pigmentosa/mastocytosis

Wrist drop
Radial nerve lesion: trauma (e.g. secondary to a prolonged period of abnormal posture of the upper arm)

Mononeuritis multiplex *See* Mononeuritis multiplex

C7 root lesion